Weaver
Koehler

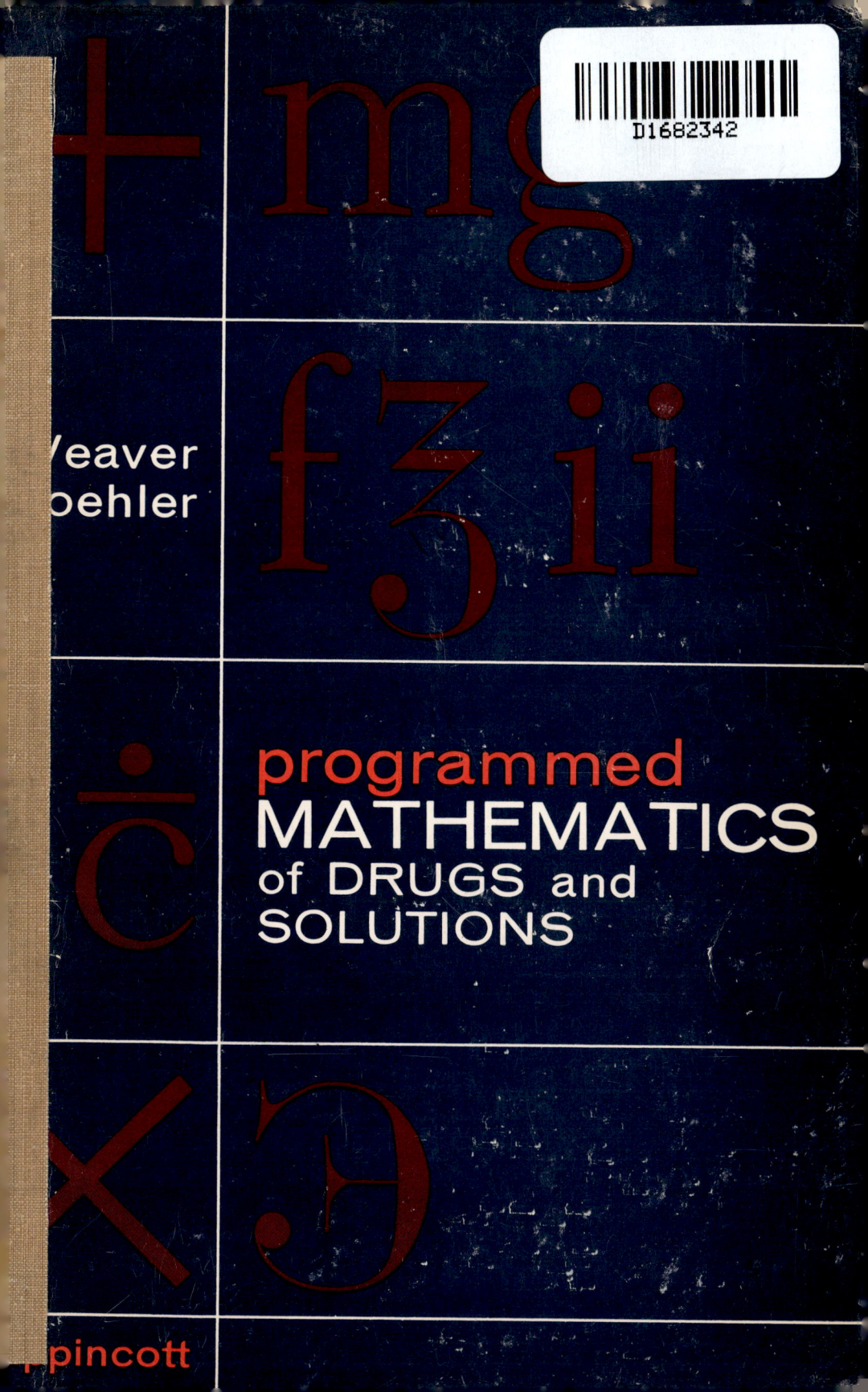

programmed
MATHEMATICS
of DRUGS and SOLUTIONS

Lippincott

programmed MATHEMATICS of DRUGS and SOLUTIONS

MABEL E. WEAVER, R.N., M.S.
Assistant Professor, Department of Nursing
Sacramento State College
Sacramento, California

VERA J. KOEHLER, R.N., M.N.
Assistant Professor, Department of Nursing
Sacramento State College
Sacramento, California

1966 REVISION WITH PEDIATRIC DOSAGES

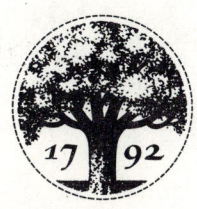

J. B. LIPPINCOTT COMPANY

Philadelphia   **Toronto**

Copyright © 1963, 1964, 1966 by Mabel E. Weaver and Vera J. Koehler. All rights reserved — no part of this material may be reproduced in any form without permission in writing from the authors.

Library of Congress Catalog Card

Number 64-66163

Printed in the United States of America

Fifth Printing

Preface

This text is designed for beginning students of nursing as a means of introducing them to the mathematics of drugs and solutions. As the volume of subject matter necessary for a nurse to master increases and class enrollments expand, the teacher-student contact time becomes more precious. Methods other than lecture-discussion which will result in as much or more learning and also provide for more efficient use of class time are being explored. Programmed texts are gaining recognition as one solution to this problem.

The authors have observed that nursing students have difficulty transferring their basic knowledge of mathematics to the content area of drugs and solutions. To find a means by which this need can be facilitated effectively and efficiently was the basis for the evolution of this text.

A basic assumption regarding arithmetic per se has been made by the authors: schools of nursing have varied mathematics requirements for admission, but these will generally include mathematics through one year of algebra. Therefore, nursing students have had courses in the basic mathematical concepts and now must be concerned with the application of these concepts to the content area of drugs and solutions. Rather than reviewing basic arithmetic as a segregated unit, the authors have incorporated this within the content of the program. Thus, the students' learning is channeled toward an area of higher motivation, that of the application of arithmetical concepts to the administration of drugs and solutions, rather than a review of arithmetic in no practical context.

Practice problems are incorporated within the book so that the student will have a frequent means of measuring progress. A comprehensive multiple choice test is also included, which the teacher may choose to use as a pre- and/or post-evaluative device.

This 50 item multiple choice test was used as the evaluative tool for determining the effectiveness of this programmed text as a teaching device. Prior to any instruction related to the mathematics of drugs and solutions, the students in two schools of nursing were given this test. Error rate on most items was high with the average number of items correct being 23. Following completion of the programmed text, some 5 months later, the students repeated this test. Error rate dropped considerably with the average number of items correct rising to 46.

Gain ratio, which is the ratio of gain actually achieved as compared with total possible gain, was computed for each student. The gain ratio

iii

score provided a measure of how much was actually taught via the program as compared with how much could be taught. The advantage of using a gain ratio score was that it takes into account the students' initial level of performance as well as their post-programmed text achievement, thus providing a measure of the effectiveness of this programmed text. The mean gain ratio of the students tested was 0.85, which means that the students learned 85 percent of what they could have possibly learned, quite a substantial gain.

Because programs are simple to use, the student can progress with considerable independence of the instructor. In fact, the better student may need no instructor — only supervised practice — after the program has been completed and the student tested with satisfactory and reliable results.

Upon completion of this program, the student should be able (1) to write the conversions of equivalents within and between the metric, the apothecary and the household systems of measurement as related to drugs and solutions, and (2) to solve problems related to drugs and solution dosages including the utilization of conversions of the metric, the apothecary and the household systems. A test which the student or the teacher may use to check student ability to meet these objectives after completing the program is included as an integral part of the text.

To the nursing students at Sacramento State College and the University of California, San Francisco, we express our appreciation for testing this programmed text. We are grateful to Miss Marjorie L. Pirie, independent study advisor at the University of California, San Francisco, for support in the initial programming and Dr. John P. DeCecco, San Francisco State College, for his critique of the programming of the chapters dealing with hypodermic tablets and injectable liquids. To the Western Council on Higher Education for Nursing Seminars on New Teaching Techniques and Dr. Henry C. Ellis, the University of New Mexico, we are grateful for expert criticism of the text and a framework for evaluating the effectiveness of the program as a teaching tool. Our appreciation is also due to our colleagues at Sacramento State College, the Fundamentals of Nursing Department, the University of California, San Francisco, family and friends who have been supportive during the development and testing of this programmed text. We are indebted to Mr. David T. Miller, Editor, Nursing Education, J.B. Lippincott Company, for his patient assistance during the preparation for publication.

MABEL E. WEAVER
VERA J. KOEHLER

CONTENTS

CHAPTER 1 The Metric System 3

CHAPTER 2 The Apothecaries' System 9

CHAPTER 3 Household Measurements 15

CHAPTER 4 Equivalents 19

CHAPTER 5 Oral Medications 31

CHAPTER 6 Hypodermic Tablets 38

CHAPTER 7 Injectable Liquids........................ 49

CHAPTER 8 Drugs Measured in Units 57

CHAPTER 9 Preparation of Drugs Packaged in Dry Form...64

CHAPTER 10 Preparation of Solutions................... 69

CHAPTER 11 Medications for Infants and Children 84

Comprehensive Examination 95

To the Student

As a part of your education, you will be learning about the administration of drugs and solutions to patients. In order to provide a person with the exact amount or dosage of medication prescribed by the physician, you, the nurse, may need to do some mathematical calculations; i.e., the drug you have available may be stated in a different system of measurement or it may be more or less than the amount that has been ordered. To assist you in learning how to solve such problems is the goal of this textbook.

In school, you studied the concepts of basic arithmetic. Now, they will take on a new meaning because you will be applying them to the preparation of drugs and solutions. Mathematical concepts which you will be using are presented in practical use within the text.

You will find names of drugs which are commonly used as medications in the problem examples. You will learn about the drugs and the actual techniques of administering them in your classes in Fundamentals, Pharmacology and Medical-Surgical Nursing, and in your clinical experience. This textbook is concerned solely with helping you to learn about the mathematics involved in drug usage. The need for accuracy in solving problems related to drugs and solutions cannot be overemphasized. As a nurse, the responsibility for accuracy is yours!

This is a programmed textbook. It is different from books you have used in the past in that the text is incomplete and is broken down into small units called frames, arranged in logical sequence. You, yourself, will complete the text by filling in words or phrases or by answering questions. You will check each answer as soon as you have written it by comparing it with the correct answer, which is found in the column to the left and below the frame you have just read.

As you work through the program, use a ruler or a strip of paper to cover the answer column. To adapt an old phrase, "The hand is quicker than the eye," we can say here that "The eye is quicker than the will power not to look."

Reading the answer is not the same as writing it yourself. It is preferable to write your answers on something other than the pages of the programmed text because it probably will be necessary for you to rework certain chapters. You need not be concerned if you make a mistake in the program as long as you rectify it. Check the correct answer and then reread the frame you missed.

With the guidance of this programmed text, you will gradually build up a vitally important body of knowledge, one step at a time. We wish you all success.

THE AUTHORS

1

The Metric System

The first step in learning about the mathematics of drugs and solutions is to become familiar with the various systems and units used in measuring drugs and solutions. First, let us consider the metric system of weights and measures. This system was developed in France in the latter part of the 18th century, and is the one presently used in most European countries. Today the metric system is being employed with increasing frequency in hospitals throughout the United States. You have become familiar with this system in various science classes. In the metric system, fractional quantities (i.e., less than one) are expressed as decimals. For example, one-half is written as 0.5.

In this system the unit of length is the meter (hence "metric"). The units which a nurse will use in measuring medications are: (1) by weight—the kilogram, the gram and the milligram, (2) by volume — the liter and the milliliter or the cubic centimeter. (Although the milliliter and the cubic centimeter are not exactly equal, the difference is so slight that the terms are used interchangeably.)

Now let us examine the relationships between these units for weight and for volume, and learn how quantities are expressed within the framework of the metric system.

1. When administering medications to her patient, the nurse will use one of three systems of measurement. The first of these that we will discuss is the international decimal system called the <u>metric</u> <u>system</u>. The ____ ____ is the international decimal system of weights and measures.

1. metric system	2. In the metric system, fractions are expressed as decimals. In the decimal system, the fraction one-half is written as 0.5. Four-tenths is written as ____.
2. 0.4	3. The unit of weight in the metric system is expressed in terms of the gram (Gm.). The _____ is said to be the unit of weight in the metric system.
3. gram	4. In the metric system, five grams is written 5.0 grams or 5.0 Gm. Ten grams is written 10.0 Gm. or ____ ____ .
4. 10.0 grams	5. The prefix "Kilo" indicates 1,000.0. A kilogram (Kg.) is _____ grams.
5. 1,000.0	6. To change kilograms to grams, <u>multiply</u> the number of kilograms by <u>1,000</u> or move the decimal three places to the <u>right</u>. Thus: 5.0 kilograms (Kg.) X 1,000 = 5,000.0 grams (Gm.) or 5.0 kilograms (Kg.) = 5.000 = 5,000.0 grams (Gm.) 10.0 Kg. = ____ Gm.
6. 10,000.0	7. 400.0 Kg. = 400,000.0 Gm. 25.0 Kg. = _____ Gm.
7. 25,000.0	8. 2.0 Kg. = _____ Gm.
8. 2,000.0	9. To change grams to kilograms, <u>divide</u> the number of grams by <u>1,000</u> or move the decimal three places to the <u>left</u>. Thus: 1,000.0 Gm. ÷ 1,000 = 1.0 Kg. or 1,000.0 Gm. = 1.000.0 = 1.0 Kg. 4,000.0 Gm. = ____ Kg.
9. 4.0	10. 60.0 Gm. = 0.06 Kg. 75.0 Gm. = ____ Kg.
10. 0.075	11. 750.0 Gm. = ____ Kg.

11. 0.75	12. The prefix <u>milli</u> indicates one one-thousandth of the unit. A milligram (mg.) is ___ _____ Gm.
12. one one-thousandth	13. One one-thousandth gram may also be written _____ Gm.
13. 0.001	14. 4.0 mg. = 0.004 Gm. 13.0 mg. = _____ Gm.
14. 0.013	15. 230.0 mg. = _____ Gm.
15. 0.23	16. To change grams to milligrams, <u>multiply</u> the number of grams by 1,000 or move the decimal three places to the <u>right</u>. Thus: 3.0 Gm. X 1,000 = 3,000.0 mg. or 3.0 Gm. = 3.<u>000</u> = 3,000.0 mg. 2.0 Gm. = ____ mg.
16. 2,000.0	17. 15.0 Gm. = 15,000.0 mg. 35.0 Gm. = _____ mg.
17. 35,000.0	18. 1.5 Gm. = _____ mg.
18. 1,500.0	19. To change milligrams to grams, <u>divide</u> the number of milligrams by 1,000 or move the decimal three places to the <u>left</u>. Thus: 1,200.0 mg. ÷ 1,000 = 1.2 Gm. or 1,200.0 mg. = 1.200.0 = 1.2 Gm. 50.0 mg. = _____ Gm.
19. 0.05	20. 14.0 mg. = 0.014 Gm. 100.0 mg. = _____ Gm.
20. 0.10	21. 250.0 mg. = _____ Gm.

21. 0.25	22. Volume in the metric system is expressed in terms of the <u>liter</u> (L.). The _____ is the unit of volume in the metric system.
22. liter	23. The nurse will most frequently use the liter (L.) and the <u>milliliter</u> (ml.). You will recall that the prefix <u>milli</u> means one one-thousandth of a unit. Here the prefix <u>milli</u> indicates the ___ _____ part of a liter.
23. one one-thousandth	24. One <u>milliliter</u> (ml.) and one <u>cubic centimeter</u> (cc.) are considered equivalent. Therefore, 10.0 ml. and _____ cc. can be used interchangeably.
24. 10.0	25. To change liter (L.) to milliliters (ml.), <u>multiply</u> the number of liters by 1,000 or move the decimal three places to the <u>right</u>. Thus: 2.0 L. X 1,000 = 2,000.0 ml. (or cc.) or 2.0 L. = 2.000 = 2,000.0 ml. (or cc.) 10.0 L. = _____ ml. (or cc.)
25. 10,000.0	26. 15.0 L. = 15,000.0 ml. (or cc.) 33.0 L. = _____ ml. (or cc.)
26. 33,000.0	27. 4.0 L. = _____ ml. (or cc.)
27. 4,000.0	28. To change milliliters (or cubic centimeters) to liters, <u>divide</u> the number of milliliters by 1,000 or move the decimal three places to the <u>left</u>. Thus: 1,500.0 ml. ÷ 1,000 = 1.5 L. or 1,500.0 ml. = 1.500.0 = 1.5 L. 15.0 cc. = _____ L.
28. 0.015	29. 18.0 cc. = 0.018 L. 250.0 cc. = _____ L.
29. 0.25	30. 965.0 cc. = _____ L.

30. 0.965

31. Following are a few problems to review what you have just learned.

PRACTICE PROBLEMS
METRIC SYSTEM
(ANSWERS ON PAGE 8)

A. 0.25 L. = _____ ml.

B. 4.0 L. = _____ ml.

C. 500.0 ml. = _____ L.

D. 1,320.0 ml. = _____ L.

E. 8.0 mg. = _____ Gm.

F. 750.0 mg. = _____ Gm.

G. 10.0 Gm. = _____ mg.

H. 3.0 Gm. = _____ mg.

I. 154.0 cc. = _____ L.

J. 1.75 L. = _____ cc.

ANSWERS TO PROBLEMS ON PAGE 7
METRIC SYSTEM

A. 250.0

B. 4,000.0

C. 0.5

D. 1.32

E. 0.008

F. 0.75

G. 10,000.0

H. 3,000.0

I. 0.154

J. 1,750.0

2

The Apothecaries' System

The apothecaries' system is the system of weights and measures which has been traditionally used in the United States to dispense drugs. This system dates back to early Colonial days, and was part of the system of weights and measures then in use in England. At that time, the unit "grain" was considered the weight of a grain of wheat, and the "minim" was the quantity of water equal to the weight of a grain of wheat. You will find the apothecaries' system in use in hospitals throughout the United States today. In some hospitals it is used exclusively, and in others it is used in combination with the metric system.

Units of weight of the apothecaries' system used to measure drugs are the grain, the dram and the ounce. Fluid volume is measured by the minim, the fluidram, the fluidounce, the pint and the quart. The terms fluidram and fluidounce are usually shortened to dram and ounce with the understanding that drugs in liquid form would be measured by volume and those in solid form would be measured by weight.

As you work through this chapter you will learn the proper notation for this system and the relationships between the various units.

	1. The second system we will consider is the <u>apothecaries' system</u>. This was the original system used in the United States. In medicine today the apothecaries' system is largely being replaced by the metric system. However, it is important for the nurse to understand both the metric and the _____ systems.

9

1. apothecaries'	2. In the apothecaries' system, quantities less than one are expressed as common fractions. One-tenth is written 1/10. Therefore, three-fourths is written _____.
2. 3/4	3. An exception to this rule is the frequent writing of one-half as $\overline{ss}$ (Latin "semis"). One-half is written 0.5, $\overline{ss}$. (Select the correct answer.)
3. $\overline{ss}$ is correct.	4. Notations in the apothecaries' system use lower case Roman numerals: i (1), v (5), x (10), 1 (50), c (100). Five and one-half is written v$\overline{ss}$. One and one-half is written _____.
4. i$\overline{ss}$	5. Seven and one-half is written _____.
5. vii$\overline{ss}$	6. Mixed numbers other than those containing one-half are written as 3 3/4. Therefore, two and one-fourth would be written _____.
6. 2 1/4	7. Arabic numerals are used in working problems in the apothecaries' system rather than lower case Roman numerals. When working problems in the apothecaries' system, _____ numerals are used.
7. Arabic	8. The most commonly used unit for weight of medications in the apothecaries' system is the <u>grain</u> (gr.). The unit of measure is placed before the numeral: five grains is written grains v or gr. v. ten grains is written _____ or _____.
8. grains x gr. x	9. Six and one-half grains is written _____ or _____.

9. grains vi$\overline{ss}$ gr. vi$\overline{ss}$	10. 1/200 of a grain is written _____ .
10. grains 1/200 or gr. 1/200	11. Volume in the apothecaries' system is expressed as minims (m.), drams (ʒ), ounce (℥), pint (pt.) and quart (qt.) minims (m.) lx (60) = drams (ʒ)i minims (m.) cxx(120) = drams (ʒ) ___ .
11. ii	12. drams (ʒ) iii = minims (m.) (clxxx). drams (ʒ) iv = minims (m.) _____ .
12. ccxl (240)	13. Using notations as for working of problems: ʒ 2 = m. _____
13. 120	14. ʒ 8 = ounce (℥) 1 Therefore, ʒ 32 = ℥ _____
14. 4	15. ʒ 40 = ℥ 5 ʒ 20 = ℥ _____
15. 2 1/2	16. ℥ 2 = ʒ 16 ℥ 3 = ʒ _____
16. 24	17. ℥ 6 = ʒ _____
17. 48	18. There are 16 ounces in one pint (pt.). ℥ 16 = pt. 1 ℥ 8 = pt. _____
18. 1/2	19. ℥ 32 = pt. _____
19. 2	20. pt. 3 = ℥ 48 pt. 5 = ℥ _____
20. 80	21. pt. 10 = ℥ _____

21. 160	22. There are two pints in one quart (qt.). pt. 2 = qt. 1 pt. 4 = qt. _____
22. 2	23. pt. 3 = qt. _____
23. 1 1/2	24. qt. 6 = pt. 12 qt. 12 = pt. _____
24. 24	25. qt. 2 1/2 = pt. _____
25. 5	

PRACTICE PROBLEMS
APOTHECARIES' SYSTEM
(ANSWERS ON PAGE 14)

A. ℥ iv$\overline{ss}$ = ℥ _____

B. ℈ viii = ℥ _____

C. m. lx = ℨ _____

D. ℨ xii = ℥ _____

E. pt. $\overline{ss}$ = ℨ _____

F. qt. 2 = pt. _____

G. m. xxx = ℨ _____

H. pt. vi = qt. _____

I. ℥ viii = ℈ _____

J. ℨ iv = m. _____

**SEE OTHER SIDE
FOR ANSWERS**

ANSWERS TO PROBLEMS ON PAGE 12
APOTHECARIES' SYSTEM

A. 36	E. 8	H. 3
B. 1	F. 4	I. 64
C. 1	G. $\overline{ss}$ (1/2)	J. 240
D. 1 1/2		

3

Household Measurements

    Household measurements are those commonly used in everyday home situations. You will recognize these measurements as those you have used in following recipes and shopping in the supermarket. Household measurements are not as accurate as those of the metric and the apothecaries' systems and, therefore, are not used to pour medications when either of the other systems is available. If you will examine spoons, cups and glasses in your own home, it will be evident to you that there is considerable variation in capacity. You, as a nurse, may find that the household measurement may be the only one you have to go by when working in a home situation. These are measurements with which the patient is familiar, and there are situations in which they may be used with safety; e.g., "normal saline solution" for a gargle.

1. Household measurements are not as accurate as metric or apothecaries' system measurements and therefore are not used as frequently in medicine. However, the nurse in the home often will find accurate measures not available and must use what she has. Household measures are not as desirable as metric or apothecaries' measures because they are less _____.

1. accurate	2. <u>Sixty</u> <u>drops</u> (gtt.) is considered <u>one</u> teaspoonful (t.). 60 gtt. (drops) = 1 t. (teaspoonful) Therefore, 120 gtt. = _____ t.
2. 2	3. 5 t. = 300 gtt. 3 t. = ___ gtt.
3. 180	4. 30 gtt. = ____ t.
4. 1/2	5. <u>Four</u> <u>teaspoonfuls</u> (t.) equal <u>one</u> tablespoonful (T.). 4 t. (teaspoonfuls) = 1 T. (tablespoonful) 8 t. = _____ T.
5. 2	6. 6 T. = 24 t. 4 T. = ____ t.
6. 16	7. 10 t. = _____ T.
7. 2 1/2	8. <u>Two</u> <u>tablespoonfuls</u> (T.) equal <u>one</u> <u>fluid</u> <u>ounce</u>. 2 T. = 1 ounce (the word fluid is usually omitted) 4 T. = _____ ounces.
8. 2	9. 5 ounces = 10 T. 4 ounces = _____ T.
9. 8	10. 12 T. = _____ ounces.
10. 6	11. <u>Six</u> <u>fluid</u> <u>ounces</u> equal <u>one</u> <u>cupful</u>. 6 ounces = 1 cupful (or teacupful) 12 ounces = _____ cupfuls.
11. 2	12. 10 cupfuls = 60 ounces. 3 cupfuls = _____ ounces.

12. 18	13. 48 ounces = _____ cupfuls.
13. 8	14. <u>Eight fluid ounces equal one glassful.</u> 8 ounces = 1 glassful 16 ounces = _____ glassfuls.
14. 2	15. 7 glassfuls = 56 ounces 4 glassfuls = ____ ounces.
15. 32	16. 24 ounces = _____ glassfuls.
16. 3	17. <u>Two pints (pt.) equal one quart (qt.)</u> 2 pt. (pints) = 1 qt. (quart). Therefore, 4 pt. = _____ qt.
17. 2	18. 5 qt. = 10 pt. 3 qt. = ____ pt.
18. 6	19. 10 qt. = ____ pt.
19. 20	

PRACTICE PROBLEMS
HOUSEHOLD MEASUREMENTS
(ANSWERS ON PAGE 18)

A. 3 T. = _____ ounces

B. 5 ounces = _____ T.

C. 6 cupfuls = _____ ounces

D. 4 quarts = _____ pints

E. 6 t. = _____ T.

F. 12 ounces = _____ glassfuls

G. 3 glassfuls = _____ ounces

H. 3 cupfuls = _____ ounces

I. 3 T. = ____ t.

J. 4 t. = _____ gtt.

ANSWERS TO PROBLEMS ON PAGE 17
HOUSEHOLD MEASUREMENTS

A. 1 1/2   F. 1 1/2

B. 10   G. 24

C. 36   H. 18

D. 8   I. 12

E. 1 1/2   J. 240

4

Equivalents

By definition, an equivalent is a given quantity which is considered to be of equal value to a quantity that is expressed in a different system. In comparing the metric, the apothecaries' and the household systems, you will find that a unit of one system never exactly equals a unit of another system; i.e., one ounce is exactly 29.5729 grams. In working problems of dosage, you will round off to the nearest whole number; hence, 30.0 grams is the approximate equivalent of one ounce. By using the approximate equivalent in computation, you would obtain a slightly different answer than if you used the exact equivalent; however, a difference of 10 percent or less is considered legitimate.

Because these three systems of weights and measures are currently in use in the United States, it is most important that you not only thoroughly understand each of the systems, but that you be able to convert from one to another accurately and without hesitation.

At the end of this chapter you will find a list of approximate equivalents which are considered a basic part of every nurse's knowledge.

	1. As you may have begun to suspect, there will be times when you will have to use the three measurement systems you have just studied interchangeably. The order for the drug may be in metric terms, and the method of measurement available in _____ or _____ systems.

19

1. apothecaries' household	2. An equivalent is an amount in one system which may be substituted for a like amount in another system. However, the _____ may not be exactly equal to the original measure.
2. equivalent	3. For example: 1.0 Gm. is exactly equal to 15.432 grains. In computing dosages of medications, however, the nurse will substitute 15 grains for 1.0 gram when necessary. We can say that grains 15 is the _____ of 1.0 gram.
3. equivalent	4. When it is necessary to convert from one system to another, it doesn't matter if the desired dose or the on-hand dose is the one which is converted. Most nurses find it simpler to convert the desired dose to that on hand; therefore, in this text we will convert the _____ _____ to the dose on hand.
4. desired dose	5. To change <u>grams</u> to <u>grains</u>, multiply the number of grams by 15. grams X 15 = _____ .
5. grains	6. Example: How many grains are in 2.0 grams? grams X 15 = grains 2.0 grams X 15 = grains _____ .
6. 30	7. Example: 0.5 Gm. is how many grains? 0.5 Gm. X 15 = gr. _____ .
7. 7 1/2	Note: In this chapter, you will find practice problems for each type of conversion immediately following the explanatory frames. An over-all problem review will be found at the end of the chapter.

PRACTICE PROBLEMS
GRAMS TO GRAINS
(ANSWERS ON PAGE 28)

A. 30.0 Gm. = gr. _____   D. 0.05 Gm. = gr. _____

B. 32.0 Gm. = gr. _____   E. 0.1 Gm. = gr. _____

C. 3.0 Gm. = gr. _____

---

	8. To change <u>grains</u> to <u>grams</u>, divide the number of grains by 15. grains ÷ 15 = _____ .
8. grams	9. Example: 45 grains is how many grams? grains ÷ 15 = grams gr. 45 ÷ 15 = _____ grams
9. 3.0	10. Example: grains 5 is what part of a gram? gr. 5 ÷ 15 = _____ grams
10. 0.3	

PRACTICE PROBLEMS
GRAINS TO GRAMS
(ANSWERS ON PAGE 28)

A. gr. i = _____ Gm.   D. gr. iii = _____ Gm.

B. gr. v = _____ Gm.   E. gr. 1/4 = _____ Gm.

C. gr. 3 3/4 = _____ Gm.

---

	11. In computing dosages of medications, 30.0 grams is considered the equivalent of ℥ i. Therefore, we can say _____ Gm. is ℥ i .
11. 30.0	12. To change <u>grams</u> to <u>ounces</u>, divide the number of grams by 30. grams ÷ 30 = _____

12. ounces	13. Example: In 60.0 grams there are how many ounces? grams ÷ 30 = ounces 60.0 Gm. ÷ 30 = ounces _____
13. 2	14. Example: How many ounces are in 150.0 grams? 150.0 Gm. ÷ 30 = ounces _____
14. 5	

PRACTICE PROBLEMS
GRAMS TO OUNCES
(ANSWERS ON PAGE 28)

A. 30.0 Gm. = ℥ _____   D. 70.0 Gm. = ℥ _____

B. 15.0 Gm. = ℥ _____   E. 90.0 Gm. = ℥ _____

C. 135.0 Gm. = ℥ _____

	15. To change <u>ounces</u> to <u>grams</u>, multiply the number of ounces by 30. ounces × 30 = _____
15. grams	16. Example: How many grams are in 4 ounces? ounces × 30 = grams ℥ 4 × 30 = _____ grams
16. 120.0	17. Example: How many grams are in ounces vi$\overline{ss}$? ℥ 6 1/2 × 30 = _____ grams
17. 195.0	

PRACTICE PROBLEMS
OUNCES TO GRAMS
(ANSWERS ON PAGE 28)

A. ℥ iii = _____ Gm. D. ℥ lxi = _____ Gm.

B. ℥ vii = _____ Gm. E. ℥ xl = _____ Gm.

C. ℥ xx = _____ Gm.

	18. 30.0 cc. is considered the equivalent of ℥ i. In converting from metric to apothecaries' systems the nurse will consider ___ cc. as being equal to ℥ i.
18. 30.0	19. To change <u>cc.</u> to <u>ounces</u>, divide the number of cc. by 30. cc. ÷ 30 = _____
19. ounces	20. Example: 240.0 cc. is how many ounces? cc. ÷ 30 = ounces 240.0 cc. ÷ 30 = ℥ _____
20. 8	21. Example: How many ounces are there in 180.0 cc.? 180.0 cc. ÷ 30 = ℥ _____
21. 6	

PRACTICE PROBLEMS
CUBIC CENTIMETERS TO OUNCES
(ANSWERS ON PAGE 29)

A. 40.0 cc. = ℥ _____   D. 1,000.0 cc. = ℥ _____

B. 60.0 cc. = ℥ _____   E. 80.0 cc. = ℥ _____

C. 105.0 cc. = ℥ _____

	22. To change <u>ounces</u> to <u>cc.</u> multiply the number of ounces by 30. ounces X 30 = _____
22. cc.	23. Example: A four-ounce bottle holds how many cc.? ounces X 30 = cc. ℥ 4 X 30 = ___ cc.
23. 120.0	24. Example: How many cc. are in 10 ounces? ℥ 10 X 30 = _____ cc.
24. 300.0	

PRACTICE PROBLEMS
OUNCES TO CUBIC CENTIMETERS
(ANSWERS ON PAGE 29)

A. ℥ ii = ___ cc. D. ℥ iiss = ___ cc.

B. ℥ vi = ___ cc. E. ℥ xv = ___ cc.

C. ℥ xxx = ___ cc.

	25. In working problems, 1.0 cc. is equivalent to minims xv. Therefore, 1.0 cc. may be substituted for m.____ .
25. 15	26. To change <u>cc.</u> to <u>minims</u>, multiply the number of cc. by 15. cc. X 15 = _____
26. minims	27. Example: In 15.0 cc. there are how many minims? cc. X 15 = minims 15.0 cc. X 15 = m. _____

27. 225	28. Example: How many minims are in 5 cubic centimeters? 5.0 cc. X 15 = m. ____
28. 75	

PRACTICE PROBLEMS
CUBIC CENTIMETERS TO MINIMS
(ANSWERS ON PAGE 29)

A. 3.0 cc. = m. ____   D. 7.0 cc. = m. ____

B. 1.5 cc. = m. ____   E. 2.2 cc. = m. ____

C. 10.0 cc. = m. ____

	29. To change <u>minims</u> to <u>cc.</u>, divide the number of minims by 15. minims ÷ 15 = _____
29. cc.	30. Example: How many cc. are there in 45 minims? minims ÷ 15 = cc. m. 45 ÷ 15 = ____ cc.
30. 3.0	31. Example: How would you measure 60 minims in a medicine glass marked only in cc.? m. 60 ÷ 15 = ____ cc.
31. 4.0	

PRACTICE PROBLEMS
MINIMS TO CUBIC CENTIMETERS
(ANSWERS ON PAGE 29)

A. m. xxx = ___ cc.

B. m. cl = ___ cc.

C. m. xc = ___ cc.

D. m. lxviiss = ___ cc.

E. m. v = ___ cc.

	32. The metric equivalent of gr. i is 60.0 mg. In working problems, the nurse will substitute ___ mg. for gr.i.
32. 60.0	33. To change <u>milligrams</u> to <u>grains</u>, divide the number of milligrams by 60. Milligrams ÷ 60 = _____
33. grains	34. Example: How many grains are in 600.0 mg.? milligrams ÷ 60 = grains 600.0 mg. ÷ 60 = gr. _____
34. 10	35. Example: How many grains are in 20.0 mg.? 20.0 mg. ÷ 60 = gr. _____
35. 1/3	36. Example: 10.0 mg. is how many grains? 10.0 mg. ÷ 60 = gr. _____
36. 1/6	

PRACTICE PROBLEMS
MILLIGRAMS TO GRAINS
(ANSWERS ON PAGE 29)

A. 75.0 mg. = gr. _____

B. 1,200.0 mg. = gr. _____

C. 300.0 mg. = gr. _____

D. 1.0 mg. = gr. _____

E. 0.3 mg. = gr. _____

	37. To change <u>grains</u> to <u>milligrams</u>, multiply the number of grains by 60. grains X 60 = _____
37. milligrams	38. Example: How many milligrams are in gr. xii? grains X 60 = milligrams gr. 12 X 60 = ____ mg.
38. 720.0	39. Example: How many milligrams are in gr. $\overline{ss}$? gr. 1/2 X 60 = ____ mg.
39. 30.0	40. Example: gr. ii is how many milligrams? gr. 2 X 60 = ____ mg.
40. 120.0	

PRACTICE PROBLEMS
GRAINS TO MILLIGRAMS
(ANSWERS ON PAGE 30)

A. gr. 1/30 = ____ mg.

B. gr. 1/4 = ____ mg.

C. gr. iii = ____ mg.

D. gr. 1/200 = ____ mg.

E. gr. ix = ____ mg.

REVIEW PROBLEMS
EQUIVALENTS
(ANSWERS ON PAGE 30)

A. 15.0 Gm. = gr. _____ .

B. 15.0 cc. = ℥ _____ .

C. 40.0 Gm. = ℥ _____ .

D. m. xl = _____ cc.

E. 80.0 mg. = gr. _____ .

F. ℥ xii = _____ Gm.

G. gr. iv = _____ mg.

H. gr. xi = _____ Gm.

I. ℥ vii$\overline{ss}$ = _____ cc.

J. 20.0 cc. = m. _____ .

ANSWERS TO PROBLEMS ON PAGE 21
GRAMS TO GRAINS

A. grams X 15 = grains
   30.0 Gm. X 15 = gr. 450

B. 32.0 Gm. X 15 = gr. 480

C. 3.0 Gm. X 15 = gr. 45

D. 0.05 Gm. X 15 =
   gr. 0.75 = gr. 3/4

E. 0.1 Gm. X 15 = gr. 1.5 =
   gr. 1 1/2

ANSWERS TO PROBLEMS ON PAGE 21
GRAINS TO GRAMS

A. grains ÷ 15 = grams
   gr. 1 ÷ 15 = 0.066 Gm.

B. gr. 5 ÷ 15 = 0.3 Gm.

C. gr. 3 3/4 ÷ 15 =
   gr. 3.75 ÷ 15 = 0.25 Gm.

D. gr. 3 ÷ 15 = 0.2 Gm.

E. gr. 1/4 ÷ 15 =
   gr. 0.25 ÷ 15 = 0.016 Gm.

ANSWERS TO PROBLEMS ON PAGE 22
GRAMS TO OUNCES

A. grams ÷ 30 = ounces
   30.0 Gm. ÷ 30 = ℥ 1

B. 15.0 Gm. ÷ 30 = ℥ 0.5 =
   ℥ 1/2

C. 135.0 Gm. ÷ 30 = ℥ 4 1/2

D. 70.0 Gm. ÷ 30 = ℥ 2 1/3

E. 90.0 Gm. ÷ 30 = ℥ 3

ANSWERS TO PROBLEMS ON PAGE 23
OUNCES TO GRAMS

A. ounces X 30 = grams
   ℥ 3 X 30 = 90.0 Gm.

B. ℥ 7 X 30 = 210.0 Gm.

C. ℥ 20 X 30 = 600.0 Gm.

D. ℥ 61 X 30 = 1,830.0 Gm.

E. ℥ 40 X 30 = 1,200.0 Gm.

ANSWERS TO PROBLEMS ON PAGE 23
CUBIC CENTIMETERS TO OUNCES

A. cc. ÷ 30 = ounces
   40.0 cc. ÷ 30 = ℥ 1 1/3

B. 60.0 cc. ÷ 30 = ℥ 2

C. 105.0 cc. ÷ 30 = ℥ 3 1/2

D. 1000.0 cc. ÷ 30 = ℥ 33 1/3

E. 80.0 cc. ÷ 30 = ℥ 2 2/3

ANSWERS TO PROBLEMS ON PAGE 24
OUNCES TO CUBIC CENTIMETERS

A. ounces X 30 = cc.
   ℥ 2 X 30 = 60.0 cc.

B. ℥ 6 X 30 = 180.0 cc.

C. ℥ 30 X 30 = 900.0 cc.

D. ℥ 2 1/2 X 30 = 75.0 cc.

E. ℥ 15 X 30 = 450.0 cc.

ANSWERS TO PROBLEMS ON PAGE 25
CUBIC CENTIMETERS TO MINIMS

A. cc. X 15 = m.
   3.0 cc. X 15 = m. 45

B. 1.5 cc. X 15 = m. 22 1/2

C. 10.0 cc. X 15 = m. 150

D. 7.0 cc. X 15 = m. 105

E. 2.2 cc. X 15 = m. 33

ANSWERS TO PROBLEMS ON PAGE 26
MINIMS TO CUBIC CENTIMETERS

A. minims ÷ 15 = cc.
   m. 30 ÷ 15 = 2.0 cc.

B. m. 150 ÷ 15 = 10.0 cc.

C. m. 90 ÷ 15 = 6.0 cc.

D. m. 67 1/2 ÷ 15 = 4.5 cc.

E. m. 5 ÷ 15 = 0.33 cc.

ANSWERS TO PROBLEMS ON PAGE 26
MILLIGRAMS TO GRAINS

A. mg. ÷ 60 = grains
   75.0 mg. ÷ 60 = gr. 1 1/4

B. 1,200.0 mg. ÷ 60 = gr. 20

C. 300.0 mg. ÷ 60 = gr. 5

D. 1.0 mg. ÷ 60 = gr. 1/60

E. 0.3 mg. ÷ 60 = gr. 1/200

ANSWERS TO PROBLEMS ON PAGE 27
GRAINS TO MILLIGRAMS

A. grains X 60 = milligrams
   gr. 1/30 X 60 = 2.0 mg.

B. gr. 1/4 X 60 = 15.0 mg.

C. gr. 3 X 60 = 180.0 mg.

D. gr. 1/200 X 60 = 0.3 mg.

E. gr. 9 X 60 = 540.0 mg.

ANSWERS TO REVIEW PROBLEMS ON PAGE 27

A. 225

B. 1/2

C. 1 1/3

D. 2.66

E. 1 1/3

F. 360.0

G. 240.0

H. 0.73

I. 225.0

J. 300

TABLE OF APPROXIMATE EQUIVALENTS

The following approximate equivalents are those considered to be essential knowledge for all nurses. (They may not be exactly what you might calculate by the preceding methods.) This table may be used as a reference for the work to follow.

1 Kg. = 2.2 lb.	0.3 mg. = gr. 1/200
30.0 Gm. = ʒ 1	1,000.0 cc. = qt. 1
1.0 Gm. = gr. 15	250.0 cc. = ʒ 8
0.3 Gm. = gr. 5	30.0 cc. = ʒ 1
0.2 Gm. = gr. 3	4.0 cc. = ʒ 1
60.0 mg. = gr. 1	1.0 cc. = m. 15
30.0 mg. = gr. 1/2	0.6 cc. = m. 10
10.0 mg. = gr. 1/6	0.06 cc. = m. 1
1.0 mg. = gr. 1/60	0.03 cc. = m. 1/2
0.4 mg. = gr. 1/150	gtt. 1 = m. 1
	tsp. 1 = dram 1

60 m = ʒ 1

5

Oral Medications

The most commonly used method of administering medications is by mouth. This is considered the safest method and is usually the easiest for both patient and nurse. Oral medications are usually the first that you will give as a student. Medications to be given p.o. (per os — by mouth) come in varied forms: tablets, pills, capsules, powders and liquids.

The medication that you have on hand frequently will be of a different dosage from the one you desire to administer. Therefore, you will need to calculate how many or what part of this oral medication will be necessary to give your patient the correct dosage which the doctor has prescribed. Many tablets are scored so that they may easily be broken into halves or quarters. Medications that are soluble in water may be dissolved to divide the dose. Here, too, you may need to put your knowledge of equivalents to work.

	1. In preparing to administer oral medications the nurse may find that the physician has prescribed a dose which is different from the size of tablet on the medication shelf. When the size of the prescribed _____ and that of the tablets on hand are not the same, the nurse must determine how much of the medication on hand should be given.

1. dose	2. If the size of the tablet on hand is larger than the prescribed dose, less than one _____ will be needed.
2. tablet	3. If the size of the tablet on hand is smaller than the prescribed dose, _____ than one tablet will be used.
3. more	4. To calculate the part of a tablet to be used or the ___ __ _____ the nurse will use the formula given in frame 5.
4. number of tablets	5. Formula: $$\frac{\text{Desired dose}}{\text{On hand dose}} \text{ or } \frac{D}{H}$$ The desired dose (D) is the _____ of medication prescribed.
5. amount or quantity	6. To solve the formula $\frac{D}{H}$ the quantity D is _____ by the quantity H.
6. divided	7. Example: The order is for 1,000.0 mg. of a certain drug. The tablets on hand are labeled 2,000.0 mg. How much of the tablet will be used? We will work together step by step: Use the formula $\frac{D}{H}$ and substitute known values _____ $\frac{mg.}{mg.}$
7. $\frac{1,000.0}{2,000.0}$	8. $\frac{D}{H} = \frac{1,000.0 \text{ mg.}}{2,000.0 \text{ mg.}} = 1,000.0 \text{ mg.} \div 2,000.0 \text{ mg.} =$ = _____ of the 2,000.0 mg. tablet will be used.

8. 0.5	9. Another way to solve the formula $\dfrac{D}{H}$ is to reduce the fraction to its lowest terms. $\dfrac{D}{H} = \dfrac{1,000.0 \text{ mg.}}{2,000.0 \text{ mg.}} = \underline{\quad}$ of the 2,000.0 mg. tablet will be used.
9. 1/2	10. The nurse should use the method she finds easiest or may use the two _____ interchangeably.
10. methods	11. Example: the order is for Demerol (p.o.) 100.0 mg. The tablets on hand are 50.0 mg. $\dfrac{D}{H} = \dfrac{\underline{\qquad} \text{ mg.}}{\underline{\qquad} \text{ mg.}}$ Substitute known values.
11. $\dfrac{100.0}{50.0}$	12. $\dfrac{D}{H} = \dfrac{100.0 \text{ mg.}}{50.0 \text{ mg.}} = \dfrac{2}{1}$ or $\underline{\qquad}$ tablets of Demerol 50.0 mg. each will be used.
12. 2	13. Using the alternate method: $\dfrac{D}{H} = \dfrac{100.0 \text{ mg.}}{50.0 \text{ mg.}} = 100.0 \text{ mg} \div 50.0 \text{ mg} =$ _____ tablets of Demerol 50.0 mg. each will be used.
13. 2	14. The same formula may be used when oral liquids are ordered. The container will be labeled according to the amount of the drug in each cc. of the liquid. In this case the amount of drug per cc. will be the _____ of the formula $\dfrac{D}{H}$

14. H	15. Example: The label indicates that there is 1.0 Gm. of the drug in each cc. How will you give 1.5 Gm.? $\dfrac{D}{H} = \dfrac{1.5 \text{ Gm.}}{1.0 \text{ Gm./cc}} = $ ___ cc. will be given.
15. 1.5	16. Following are some problems for reviewing this material. Use either method — or both. This formula may be used with any measurement system. When two systems of measurement are involved, be sure the D and the H are in the same system.

PRACTICE PROBLEMS
ORAL MEDICATIONS
(ANSWERS ON PAGES 36-37)

1. From reserpine 0.25 mg., give 0.5 mg.

2. On hand, codeine sulfate 30.0 mg. Give 60.0 mg.

3. From terramycin 100.0 mg. per ml., give 0.3 Gm.

4. From chlorpromazine 10.0 mg. per 2.0 ml., give 0.02 Gm.

5. Gtt. 15 are ordered. How many minims is this?

6. Acetysalicylic acid gr. x has been ordered; how will you give this amount from tablets gr. iiss?

7. Give meprobamate 400.0 mg. from tablets 200.0 mg.

8. Give caffeine 0.2 Gm. from tablets gr. iii.

9. Gantrisin tablets on hand, gr. v. How will you give 1.0 Gm.?

10. How will you tell a mother to measure ℨi of a prescription to give to her child?

11. From sulfasoxazole 500.0 mg. tablets, give gr. xv.

12. Give phenobarbital gr. $\overline{ss}$ from tablets 15.0 mg.

13. How will you give atropine sulfate gr. 1/200 from tablets 0.3 mg.?

14. How can you measure 1 fluid ounce with equipment found in the home?

15. How will you give gr. 1/6 of a drug from tablets labeled 10.0 mg.?

ANSWERS TO PRACTICE PROBLEMS ON PAGES 34-35
ORAL MEDICATIONS

1. $\dfrac{D}{H} = \dfrac{0.5 \text{ mg.}}{0.25 \text{ mg.}} =$ 2 tablets of reserpine 0.25 mg. will be used.

2. $\dfrac{D}{H} = \dfrac{60.0 \text{ mg.}}{30.0 \text{ mg.}} =$ 2 tablets of codeine sulfate 30.0 mg. will be used.

3. $\dfrac{D}{H} = \dfrac{300.0 \text{ mg.}}{100.0 \text{ mg./ml.}} =$ 3.0 ml. of terramycin 100.0 mg./ml. will be used.

4. 10.0 mg. per 2.0 ml. = 5.0 mg. per 1.0 ml.

   $\dfrac{D}{H} = \dfrac{20.0 \text{ mg.}}{5.0 \text{ mg./ml.}} =$ 4.0 ml. of chlorpromazine 10.0 mg./2.0 ml. will be used.

5. 15 minims.

6. $\dfrac{D}{H} = \dfrac{\text{gr. 10}}{\text{gr. 2 1/2}} =$ 4 tablets of acetysalicylic acid gr. iiss will be given.

7. $\dfrac{D}{H} = \dfrac{400.0 \text{ mg.}}{200.0 \text{ mg.}} =$ 2 tablets of meprobamate 200.0 mg. will be given.

8. 0.2 Gm. = gr. 3

   Give 1 tablet of caffeine gr. iii.

9. 1.0 Gm. = gr. 15

   $\dfrac{D}{H} = \dfrac{\text{gr. 15}}{\text{gr. 5}} =$ 3 tablets of gantrisin gr. v will be given.

10. Use 1 teaspoonful.

11. gr. 15 = 1.0 Gm. = 1,000.0 mg.

$$\frac{D}{H} = \frac{1,000.0 \text{ mg.}}{500.0 \text{ mg.}} = \underline{2 \text{ tablets of sulfasoxazole 500.0 mg. will be given.}}$$

12. gr. s̄s̄ = 30.0 mg.

$$\frac{D}{H} = \frac{30.0 \text{ mg.}}{15.0 \text{ mg.}} = \underline{2 \text{ tablets of phenobarbital 15.0 mg. will be given.}}$$

13. 0.3 mg. = gr. 1/200

    <u>Give one tablet of atropine sulfate 0.3 mg.</u>

14. 2 tablespoonfuls.

15. 10.0 mg. = gr. 1/6

    <u>Give one tablet of drug labeled 10.0 mg.</u>

6

Hypodermic Tablets

Another route of administration for medications is the parenteral one. This refers to injecting the drug into the fluid or the tissue of the body by needle. As a nurse, you will be called on most frequently to administer medications in one of three ways: (1) intradermally — into the upper layers of the skin, (2) subcutaneously (hypodermically) — into the subcutaneous tissue of the outer surface of the upper arm or the anterior surface of the thigh, (3) intramuscularly — into the muscle tissue. In your classroom laboratory, you will have opportunity to examine various syringes and needles and you will have experience in using them.

Because some drugs will deteriorate when stored as a solution, they come from the pharmacy in the form of a small, easily dissolved tablet (although with new methods of pharmaceutical manufacturing, fewer drugs are so prepared). If the order for the drug differs from the strength you have on hand, you will use the formula presented in this chapter to determine how many tablets or what fraction of a tablet must be used to provide the correct dosage. As you work through this chapter, you will also learn how to determine the amount of diluent needed to provide the correct dose.

	1. Certain drugs come from the pharmacy in the form of small tablets designed for hypodermic use. To give a drug hypodermically one of these _____ _____ may be used.

1. small tablets	2. To prepare the drug for injection the tablet must be dissolved in a small quantity of diluent such as sterile water or sterile normal saline solution. Sterile water is the most commonly used _____.
2. diluent	3. The usual hypodermic diluent volume is between <u>10 and 20 minims.</u> This quantity is sufficient to easily dissolve the _____, and decreases the margin of error should some of the solution be lost. It is not great enough to cause discomfort to the patient from tissue distention.
3. tablet	4. To dissolve a tablet for hypodermic injection in 15 minims of sterile water would be a(an) (<u>correct, incorrect</u>) procedure.
4. correct	5. When the prescribed dose and the tablet on hand are the same, the nurse dissolves the tablet in from _____ to _____ minims of sterile water in the accepted manner. (To be demonstrated in class)
5. 10 20	6. When the prescribed dose and the tablets on hand are not the same, the nurse must determine how many tablets or what part of a _____ must be used.

6. tablet	7. You will remember that the formula to calculate the part of or the number of tablets to be used is:
	    Divide the <u>desired dose</u> by the <u>dose on hand.</u>
	This rule may also be expressed:
	    $\dfrac{\text{Desired dose}}{}$ or $\dfrac{D}{H}$

7. dose on hand	8. When the desired dose is gr. 2 and the drug on hand is labeled gr. 1, substitute in the formula and solve. $\dfrac{D}{H} = \dfrac{gr.\ 2}{gr.\ 1}$ $= 2 \div 1 =$ <u>2 tablets gr. 1 are necessary to give the desired dose of gr. 2.</u> In this formula D stands for _____. And H stands for _____.
8. desired dose dose on hand (or on hand dose)	9. Now, we will work two problems together step by step. It may help you to write out each step in full. The order on the chart reads "Give morphine sulfate gr. 1/4 q4h." The morphine sulfate which is in the narcotics cupboard is labeled gr. 1/2. $\dfrac{D}{H} = \dfrac{gr.\ 1/4}{gr.\ \underline{}}$
9. 1/2	10. $\dfrac{D}{H} = \dfrac{\cancel{gr.}\ 1/4}{\cancel{gr.}\ 1/2}$ _____
10. 1/4 ÷ 1/2	11. $\dfrac{D}{H} = \dfrac{\cancel{gr.}\ 1/4}{\cancel{gr.}\ 1/2} =$ 1/4 ÷ 1/2 = _____
11. 1/4 X 2/1 Did you remember that to divide fractions you invert the denominator and then multiply? If you did, good! If you didn't---- THINK!!!	12. $\dfrac{D}{H} = \dfrac{\cancel{gr.}\ 1/4}{\cancel{gr.}\ 1/2} =$ 1/4 ÷ 1/2 = 1/4 X 2/1 = <u>1/2 of a</u> _____ <u>of morphine sulfate gr.</u> _____ <u>will be needed.</u>

12. tablet 1/2 ALWAYS LABEL YOUR ANSWER! Now, let's try another one.	13. The preoperative order is for atropine sulfate gr. 1/300. The tablets on hand are labeled gr. 1/100. $\dfrac{D}{H} = \dfrac{\text{gr. } 1/300}{\text{gr. } 1/100} =$ $1/300 \div 1/100 = \rule{2cm}{0.4pt}$ Finish calculations and label answer.
13. $1/300 \times 100/1 =$ <u>1/3 of a tablet of atropine sulfate gr. 1/100 will be needed.</u>	14. Are you able to solve these problems without difficulty?
14. If the answer is no, please go back to frame 7 and give it another try. If the answer is yes, continue to frame 15.	15. Of the examples used so far, the first required more than one of the tablets on hand. The second and the third required only part of a tablet. To divide the tablet, dissolve it in a predetermined amount of sterile water (or other diluent) and discard that portion which is not needed. The next step is to determine the amount of _____ to be used.
15. diluent	16. Formula: To prepare, dissolve the tablet on hand in the number of minims indicated by the <u>denominator</u> and give the number of minims indicated by the <u>numerator</u>. In the fraction 3/4, 3 is the _____. and 4 is the _____.
16. numerator denominator	17. When the numerator in the fraction is less than 10, both the numerator and the denominator must be <u>multiplied</u> by the smallest whole number which will bring the numerator within the 10 to 20 minim range. Thus: $3/4 \times 4/4 = \rule{2cm}{0.4pt}$

17. 12/16	18. Therefore, to give 3/4 of a tablet: 3/4 X 4/4 = 12/16 Dissolve the tablet in _____ minims diluent and give _____ minims.
18. 16 12	19. Example: We will use the last problem that we worked where the preoperative order is for atropine sulfate gr. 1/300. The tablets on hand are labeled gr. 1/100. Again, we will work together step by step. $\dfrac{D}{H} =$ _____
19. $\dfrac{\text{gr. }1/300}{\text{gr. }1/100}$	20. $\dfrac{D}{H} = \dfrac{\text{gr. }1/300}{\text{gr. }1/100} =$ _____
20. 1/300 ÷ 1/100	21. $\dfrac{D}{H} = \dfrac{\text{gr. }1/300}{\text{gr. }1/100} =$ 1/300 ÷ 1/100 = _____
21. 1/300 X 100/1	22. $\dfrac{D}{H} = \dfrac{\text{gr. }1/300}{\text{gr. }1/100} =$ 1/300 ÷ 1/100 = 1/300 X 100/1 = _____
22. <u>1/3 of a tablet of atropine sulfate gr. 1/100 will be needed to give atropine sulfate gr. 1/300.</u>	23. 1/3 tablet X 10/10 (number to bring numerator in 10-20 minim range) = ___
23. 10/30	24. Dissolve the tablet of atropine sulfate gr. 1/3 in _____ minims diluent and give _____ minims. You then have gr. 1/300 of atropine sulfate.

43

24. 30 10	25. The 1 and the 3 of the fraction 1/3 were both multiplied by 10 because 10 is the _____ (use your words) _____ .
25. smallest whole number which will give a number between 10 and 20 when multiplied by the numerator.	26. When the tablets on hand are smaller than the required dose <u>two</u> or <u>more</u> tablets will be needed. If the number of tablets required is 1 1/2, one full tablet must be used plus _____ of a second tablet.
26. 1/2	27. To prepare 1 1/2 tablets: Method A: Prepare the 1/2 tablet as if it were to be given alone. 28. 1/2 X 10/10 = 10/20 <u>Dissolve the tablet in _____ minims diluent. Discard _____ minims. Add the second tablet to the remaining _____ minims = solution containing 1 1/2 tablets.</u>

27. 20
     10
     10
  This method can be used only when certain equipment is on hand. (To be demonatrated in class).
	28. To prepare 1 1/2 tablets:
	Method B: Determine what fraction of two tablets will be required.
	$\dfrac{D}{H} = \dfrac{3/2 \text{ tablets}}{4/2 \text{ tablets}}$
	3/2 ÷ 4/2 =
	3/2 X 2/4 = 3/4 of _____ _____ will be needed.

28. two tablets	29. 3/4 X 4/4 = 12/16 Dissolve the two tablets in _____ minims diluent; give _____ minims = solution containing 1 1/2 tablets.

29. 16
    12

30. Example: The order reads: "Give atropine sulfate gr. 1/120 stat." The tablets on hand are gr. 1/150.

    Method A:

    $$\frac{D}{H} = \frac{\text{gr. } 1/120}{\text{gr. } 1/150} =$$

    1/120 ÷ 1/150 =

    1/120 X 150/1 = 5/4 = 1 1/4 tablets atropine sulfate gr. 1/150 will be needed.

    1/4 X 10/10 = 10/40

    Dissolve one tablet in _____ minims diluent. Discard _____ minims. Add second tablet to remaining _____ minims = atropine sulfate gr. 1/120.

30. 40
    30
    10

31. Method B:

    $$\frac{D}{H} = \frac{\text{gr. } 1/120}{\text{gr. } 1/150} =$$

    1/120 ÷ 1/150 =

    1/120 X 150/1 = 5/4 = 1 1/4 tablets atropine sulfate gr. 1/150 will be needed.

    H = 2 tablets each gr. 1/150 gr. = gr. 2/150

    $$\frac{D}{H} = \frac{\text{gr. } 1/120}{\text{gr. } 2/150}$$

    1/120 ÷ 2/150 =

    1/120 X 150/2 = 5/8 of two tablets gr. 1/150 will be needed.

    5/8 X 3/3 = 15/24

    Dissolve two tablets atropine sulfate gr. 1/150 in _____ minims diluent; give _____ minims = atropine sulfate gr. 1/120.

31. 24 15	32. Here are some problems for you to work. The answers are at the end of the chapter. Work as many problems as you need to make you feel comfortable with this type of problem.

PRACTICE PROBLEMS
HYPODERMIC TABLETS
(ANSWERS ON PAGES 46-47-48)

1. How will you prepare pilocarpine gr. 1/8 from tablets gr. 1/3?

2. Give strychnine gr. 1/40. The tablets on hand are gr. 1/30.

3. Give codeine phosphate gr. 1/2 from tablets gr. 1/6.

4. Give dilaudid gr. 1/24 from tablets gr. 1/64.

5. From tablets which contain 16.0 mg. morphine sulfate give 8.0 mg.

6. From tablets on hand: dilaudid 2.0 mg. Give dilaudid 3.0 mg.

7. Give phenobarbital sodium gr. 1 1/2 from tablets labeled "Phenobarbital Sodium 60.0 mg."

8. From tablets on hand atropine sulfate gr. 1/150 give atropine sulfate 0.3 mg.

ANSWERS TO PROBLEMS ON PAGE 45
HYPODERMIC TABLETS

1. $\dfrac{D}{H} = \dfrac{gr.\ 1/8}{gr.\ 1/3} =$

    $1/8 \div 1/3 =$

    $1/8 \times 3/1 =$ <u>3/8 of a tablet pilocarpine gr. 1/3 will be needed.</u>

    $3/8 \times 4/4 = 12/32$ <u>Dissolve the tablet in 32 minims diluent.</u>
    <u>Give 12 minims</u> = <u>pilocarpine gr. 1/8.</u>

2. $\dfrac{D}{H} = \dfrac{gr.\ 1/40}{gr.\ 1/30} =$

    $1/40 \div 1/30 =$

    $1/40 \times 30/1 =$ <u>3/4 of a tablet strychnine gr. 1/30 will be needed.</u>

    $3/4 \times 4/4 = 12/16$ <u>Dissolve the tablet in 16 minims diluent.</u>
    <u>Give 12 minims</u> = <u>strychnine gr. 1/40.</u>

3. $\dfrac{D}{H} = \dfrac{gr.\ 1/2}{gr.\ 1/6} =$

    $1/2 \div 1/6 =$

    $1/2 \times 6/1 =$ <u>3 tablets codeine phosphate gr. 1/6 will be needed.</u>

    <u>Dissolve in 10 to 20 minims diluent</u> = <u>codeine phosphate gr. 1/2.</u>

4. <u>Method A:</u>

    $\dfrac{D}{H} = \dfrac{gr.\ 1/24}{gr.\ 1/64} =$

    $1/24 \div 1/64 =$

    $1/24 \times 64/1 = 8/3 =$ <u>2 2/3 tablets dilaudid gr. 1/64 will be needed.</u>

    $2/3 \times 6/6 = 12/18$ Dissolve one tablet in 18 minims diluent. Discard 6 minims. Add the two tablets to the remaining 12 minims = <u>dilaudid gr. 1/24.</u>

4. Method B:

$$\frac{D}{H} = \frac{gr. \ 1/24}{gr. \ 1/64} =$$

1/24 ÷ 1/64 =

1/24 X 64/1 = 8/3 = <u>2 2/3 tablets dilaudid gr. 1/64 will be needed.</u>

H = 3 tablets each Dilaudid gr. 1/64 = gr. 3/64 Dilaudid.

$$\frac{D}{H} = \frac{gr. \ 1/24}{gr. \ 3/64} =$$

1/24 ÷ 3/64 =

1/24 X 64/3 = <u>8/9 of three tablets dilaudid gr. 1/64 will be needed.</u>

8/9 X 2/2 = 16/18 <u>Dissolve the three tablets of dilaudid gr. 1/64 in 18 minims diluent. Discard 2 minims. Give 16 minims = dilaudid gr. 1/24.</u>

5. $$\frac{D}{H} = \frac{8.0 \ mg.}{16.0 \ mg.} =$$

8 ÷ 16 = <u>1/2 tablet 16.0 mg. morphine sulfate will be needed.</u>

1/2 X 10/10 = 10/20 <u>Dissolve tablet in 20 minims diluent; give 10 minims = 8.0 mg. morphine sulfate.</u>

6. Method A:

$$\frac{D}{H} = \frac{3.0 \ mg.}{2.0 \ mg.} =$$

3 ÷ 2 = <u>1 1/2 tablets 2.0 mg. dilaudid will be needed.</u>

1/2 X 10/10 = 10/20 <u>Dissolve one tablet in 20 minims diluent. Discard 10 minims. Add second tablet to remaining 10 minims = dilaudid 3.0 mg.</u>

Method B:

$$\frac{D}{H} = \frac{3.0 \ mg.}{2.0 \ mg.} =$$

3 ÷ 2 = <u>1 1/2 tablets 2.0 mg. dilaudid will be needed.</u>

H = 2 tablets each 2.0 mg. dilaudid = 4.0 mg. dilaudid

$$\frac{D}{H} = \frac{3.0 \ mg.}{4.0 \ mg.} =$$ <u>3/4 of two tablets 2.0 mg. dilaudid will be needed.</u>

3/4 X 4/4 = 12/16 <u>Dissolve two tablets in 16 minims diluent; give 12 minims = 3.0 mg. dilaudid.</u>

7. Method A:

   60.0 mg. = gr. 1

   $\dfrac{D}{H} = \dfrac{gr.\ 1.5}{gr.\ 1}$ = 1.5 tablets 60.0 mg. phenobarbital sodium will be needed.

   1/2 X 10/10 = 10/20   Dissolve one tablet in 20 minims diluent. Discard 10 minims. Add the second tablet to the remaining 10 minims = phenobarbital sodium gr. 1 1/2.

   Method B:

   60.0 mg. = gr. 1

   $\dfrac{D}{H} = \dfrac{gr.\ 1.5}{gr.\ 1}$ = 1.5 tablets 60.0 mg. phenobarbital sodium will be needed.

   H = 2 tablets each gr. 1 phenobarbital sodium = gr. 2 phenobarbital sodium.

   $\dfrac{D}{H} = \dfrac{gr.\ 1.5}{gr.\ 2}$ = 1.5 ÷ 2 = 0.75 = 3/4 of two tablets 60.0 mg. phenobarbital sodium will be needed.

   3/4 X 4/4 = 12/16   Dissolve two tablets in 16 minims diluent; give 12 minims = phenobarbital sodium gr. 1 1/2.

8. 0.3 mg. = gr. 1/200

   $\dfrac{D}{H} = \dfrac{gr.\ 1/200}{gr.\ 1/150}$

   1/200 ÷ 1/150 =

   1/200 X 150/1 = 3/4 of a tablet gr. 1/150 atropine sulfate will be needed.

   3/4 X 4/4 = 12/16   Dissolve tablet in 16 minims diluent. Give 12 minims = 0.3 mg. atropine sulfate.

// 7

Injectable Liquids

In Chapter 6 you dealt with drugs that deteriorate when kept in solution. However, you will find that there are many drugs which may be stored safely in liquid form. These drugs are packaged in ampuls (single dose) or vials (multiple dose) and are labeled according to the amount of the drug in the ampul or in the fractional part of the vial; e.g., Meperidine Hydrochloride 50 mg. (ampul), or Meperidine Hydrochloride 50 mg./cc. (multi-dose vial).

Should the doctor's order for the medication and the drug that is available differ in dosage, you will use the formula discussed in this chapter to determine the quantity of solution to be given. Remember here, as in working all dosage problems, that two systems of weights and measures cannot be used in one problem without first converting the units to a common system.

	1. Drugs for hypodermic injection are often kept in solutions of various strengths. These drugs are packaged in <u>ampuls</u> or <u>vials</u>. An ampul holds one dose, while a vial holds more than one dose. If you have four doses packaged together, this is called a _____.

49

1. vial	2. The container will be labeled as to the <u>amount</u> <u>of</u> <u>drug</u> in the ampul or the fractional part of the vial. A vial labeled gr. 1/4 per cc. would contain gr. 1/4 of the drug in each _____ of solution.
2. cc.	3. When the prescribed dose and the label on the ampul are the same, the nurse will use _____ of the ampul. (To be demonstrated in class.)
3. all	4. You are to give 50.0 mg. of the drug. When the vial is labeled 50.0 mg. per cc. the nurse will withdraw ____ cc. of solution from the vial.
4. 1.0	5. When the prescribed dose differs from the label, the nurse must determine how much of the _____ must be used to give the prescribed dose.
5. solution	6. To determine the amount of solution required use the following formula: $$\frac{D}{H} = \frac{x}{V}$$ In this formula: D stands for _____ H stands for _____ x stands for the desired volume V stands for the volume on hand
6. desired dose dose on hand	7. The vial is labeled: "50.0 mg. per cc." Substitute in the formula $$\frac{D}{H} = \frac{x}{}$$

7. 50.0 mg./cc	8. Example:
	The vial is labeled "Morphine sulfate: minims xv = gr. 1/8."
	Give gr. 1/6.
	
	$$\frac{D}{H} = \frac{x}{V}$$
	
	$$\frac{gr.\ 1/6}{gr.\ 1/8} = \frac{x}{m.15}$$ This is an incomplete proportion and will be solved as such.
	
	1/6 : 1/8 : : x : m.15
	1/8 x = m.15 X 1/6
	1/8 x = m.5/2
	   x = m. 5/2 ÷ 1/8
	   x = m. 5/2 X 8/1
	   x = 20 _____

8. <u>minims of solution will be needed to give morphine sulfate gr. 1/6</u>	9. Example: The vial is labeled "Nalorphine: 5.0 mg. per ml." How will you give 8.0 mg. of the drug? $$\frac{D}{H} = \frac{x}{V}$$ $$\frac{8.0\ mg.}{\rule{2em}{0.4pt}} = \frac{x}{\rule{2em}{0.4pt}}$$
9. 5.0 mg. 1.0 ml.	10. $$\frac{8.0\ mg.}{5.0\ mg.} = \frac{x}{1.0\ ml.} =$$ 8 : 5 : : x : 1.0 ml. _____ finish calculations and label answer.

10. 5 x = 8.0 ml.
   x = 8.0 ml. ÷ 5
   x = <u>1.6 ml. of solution will be needed to give 8.0 mg. nalorphine.</u>
	11. If you feel that you understand the use of this formula, continue to the following practice problems. If you are not sure of yourself, please go back to frame 1 of this section and try again.

PRACTICE PROBLEMS
INJECTABLE LIQUIDS
(ANSWERS ON PAGES 54-55-56)

1. From a streptomycin solution containing 500.0 mg. in 1.0 cc., give 400.0 mg.

2. The vial on hand is labeled: "Morphine Sulfate: Minims xxx = gr. 1/8." Give gr. 1/24 of morphine sulfate.

3. From a cortisone acetate solution containing 25.0 mg. in 1.0 cc., give 90.0 mg.

4. The stock solution is labeled: "Demerol: 1.0 cc. = 50.0 mg." Give 75.0 mg. of demerol.

5. From scopolamine 0.4 mg. per ml., give gr. 1/300.

6. Give chlorpromazine 0.050 Gm. from solution labeled 25.0 mg. per ml.

7. From digitoxin 0.2 mg. per cc., give 0.3 mg.

8. Give caffeine sodium benzoate gr. 3 3/4 from solution labeled 0.5 Gm. in 2.0 cc.

**SEE OTHER SIDE
FOR ANSWERS**

ANSWERS TO PROBLEMS ON PAGE 52
INJECTABLE LIQUIDS

1. $\dfrac{D}{H} = \dfrac{x}{V}$

   $\dfrac{400.0 \text{ mg.}}{500.0 \text{ mg.}} = \dfrac{x}{1.0 \text{ cc.}}$

   400 : 500 : : x : 1.0 cc.

   500 x = 400.0 cc.

   x = 400.0 cc. ÷ 500

   x = <u>0.8 cc. of the streptomycin solution 500.0 mg. in 1.0 cc. is needed</u> to give streptomycin 400.0 mg.

2. $\dfrac{D}{H} = \dfrac{x}{V}$

   $\dfrac{\text{gr. } 1/24}{\text{gr. } 1/8} = \dfrac{x}{30 \text{ minims (m.)}}$

   1/24 : 1/8 : : x : 30 m.

   1/8 x = 1/24 X 30 m.

   1/8 x = 5/4 m.

   x = 5/4 m. ÷ 1/8

   x = 5/4 m. X 8/1

   x = <u>10 minims of the morphine sulfate solution m. xxx = gr. 1/8 is needed</u> to give morphine sulfate gr. 1/24.

3. $\dfrac{D}{H} = \dfrac{x}{V}$

   $\dfrac{90.0 \text{ mg.}}{25.0 \text{ mg.}} = \dfrac{x}{1.0 \text{ cc.}}$

   90 : 25 : : x : 1.0 cc.

   25 x = 90.0 cc.

   x = 90.0 cc. ÷ 25

   x = <u>3.6 cc. of the cortisone acetate solution 25.0 mg., per 1.0 cc. would be used</u> (given IM because of the volume) in order to give cortisone acetate 90.0 mg.

4. $\dfrac{D}{H} = \dfrac{x}{V}$

$\dfrac{75.0 \text{ mg.}}{50.0 \text{ mg.}} = \dfrac{x}{1.0 \text{ cc.}}$

75 : 50 : : x : 1.0 cc.

50 x = 75.0 cc.

x = 75.0 cc. ÷ 50

x = 1.5 cc. <u>Demerol solution 50.0 mg. per 1.0 cc. will be used in order to give Demerol 75.0 mg. (IM)</u>

5. 0.4 mg. = gr. 1/150

$\dfrac{D}{H} = \dfrac{x}{V}$

$\dfrac{\text{gr. } 1/300}{\text{gr. } 1/150} = \dfrac{x}{1.0 \text{ ml.}}$

1/300 : 1/150 : : x : 1.0 ml.

1/150 x = 1/300 ml.

x = 1/300 ml. ÷ 1/150

x = 1/300 ml. × 150/1

x = <u>0.5 ml. of scopolamine solution labeled 0.4 mg./ml. is needed to give scopolamine gr. 1/300.</u>

6. 0.050 Gm. = 50.0 mg.

$\dfrac{D}{H} = \dfrac{x}{V}$

$\dfrac{50.0 \text{ mg.}}{25.0 \text{ mg.}} = \dfrac{x}{1.0 \text{ ml.}}$

50 : 25 : : x : 1.0 ml.

25 x = 50.0 ml.

x = 50.0 ml. ÷ 25

x = <u>2.0 ml. of the chlorpromazine solution labeled 25.0 mg./ml. is needed to give chlorpromazine 0.050 Gm.</u>

7. $\dfrac{D}{H} = \dfrac{x}{V}$

   $\dfrac{0.3 \text{ mg.}}{0.2 \text{ mg.}} = \dfrac{x}{1.0 \text{ cc.}}$

   $0.3 : 0.2 :: x : 1.0$ cc.

   $0.2 x = 0.3$ cc.

   $x = 0.3$ cc. $\div$ 0.2

   $x = \underline{1.5 \text{ cc. of digitoxin solution labeled 0.2 mg./cc. would be}}$
   $\underline{\text{needed to give digitoxin 0.3 mg}}$

8. 0.5 Gm. = gr. 7 1/2

   $\dfrac{D}{H} = \dfrac{x}{V}$

   $\dfrac{\text{gr. 3.75}}{\text{gr. 7.5}} = \dfrac{x}{2.0 \text{ cc.}}$

   $3.75 : 7.5 :: x : 2.0$ cc.

   $7.5 x = 3.75 \times 2.0$ cc.

   $7.5 x = 7.5$ cc.

   $x = 7.5$ cc. $\div$ 7.5

   $x = \underline{1.0 \text{ cc. of the caffeine sodium benzoate solution labeled 0.5}}$
   $\underline{\text{Gm./2.0 cc. would be needed to give caffeine sodium ben-}}$
   $\underline{\text{zoate gr. 3 3/4.}}$

Drugs Measured in Units

The strength of certain medications is measured in units. A unit is the quantity of drug which provides a specific action. The unit is defined for each drug, and there is <u>no</u> <u>relationship</u> between the strength of a unit of one drug and a unit of another drug. You cannot compare a unit of penicillin with a unit of tetanus antitoxin.

Insulin is another example of a medication that is measured in units. It is supplied in vials labeled U20, U40, U80 or U100. This indicates the number of units of insulin in each cubic centimeter in the vial. The least complicated and most accurate way to measure insulin is to use the insulin syringe. This is a special 1.0 cc. syringe calibrated to measure insulin units rather than cubic centimeters or minims. To give 30 units of U40 insulin you would use an insulin syringe calibrated for U40 insulin, and simply measure the 30 units. Note: the calibrations on the syringe <u>must agree</u> with the strength of the insulin to be used when the dosage is to be measured in this manner.

When you do not have an insulin syringe to use to give insulin, you may measure the dose by using a tuberculin syringe or an ordinary 2.0 cc. hypodermic syringe. The quantity of insulin to be given is calculated by using the formula presented in this chapter and is measured in minims or cubic centimeters.

This formula (which is the same basic formula you have used before) may be used to calculate the dose of any drug which is measured in units.

	1. Many biologicals are supplied in vials containing a specified number of units per cubic centimeter of the solution. A vial labeled 1,500 Units per cc. would contain _____ units of the drug in each cc. of the solution.

1. 1,500	2. The potency of the unit of each product is defined by the United States Pharmocopeia. The unit may also be called a U.S.P. _____ .
2. unit	3. These drugs are ordered by the physician according to the number of _____ to be given.
3. U.S.P. units or units	4. When the vial is labeled 1,500 U.S.P. units (or 1,500 units) per cc., the nurse will withdraw _____ cc. of solution to give 1,500 units.
4. 1.0 cc.	5. When the prescribed dose differs from what is on hand, it is the nurse's responsibility to correctly calculate how much of the _____ must be given.
5. solution	6. Again use the basic formula: $$\frac{\text{Desired dose (D)}}{\text{Dose on hand (H)}}$$ with the addition of certain words for clarity--- $$\frac{\text{Desired dose of U.S.P. Units}}{\text{Number of U.S.P. Units per cc. in Dose on hand}}$$ or $\dfrac{DU}{\underline{}}$
6. HU	7. Example: The order is for 4,500 units of tetanus antitoxin. The label on the vial is "Tetanus Antitoxin: 1,500 units per milliliter." How much solution will be needed? We will work together step by step: $$\frac{\text{Desired units}}{\text{Units on hand}} = \frac{\underline{}}{HU}$$

7. DU	8. $\dfrac{DU}{HU} = \dfrac{4{,}500 \text{ units}}{\rule{2cm}{0.4pt}}$
8. 1,500 units	9. $\dfrac{DU}{HU} = \dfrac{4{,}500 \text{ units}}{1{,}500 \text{ units per ml.}}$ $\dfrac{4{,}500}{1{,}500 \text{ ml.}} = \dfrac{3}{1.0 \text{ ml.}} = \underline{}$ of tetanus antitoxin solution containing 1,500 units per ml. will be needed to give 4,500 units of tetanus antitoxin.
9. 3.0 ml.	10. Example: Using a penicillin solution containing 100,000 units in 1.0 cc., give 40,000 units of the drug. $\dfrac{DU}{HU} = \underline{}$ Substitute values and complete calculations. Label answer.
10. $\underline{} = \dfrac{40{,}000 \text{ units}}{100{,}000 \text{ units/cc.}} =$ $\dfrac{40{,}000}{100{,}000 \text{ cc.}} = \dfrac{4}{10.0 \text{ cc.}} =$ 0.4 cc. of penicillin solution containing 100,000 units in 1.0 cc. will be needed to give 40,000 units of penicillin.	11. Next: are you ready for some practice problems?

PRACTICE PROBLEMS
DRUGS MEASURED IN UNITS
(ANSWERS ON PAGES 62-63)

1. From a vial labeled "Heparin sodium: 20,000 units per ml.," give 5,000 units of heparin sodium.

2. Give 50,000 units of sodium penicillin G from a multiple-dose vial in which 10.0 ml. contains 1,000,000 units.

3. Give penicillin 600,000 units from a solution labeled 3,000,000 units per 5.0 ml.

4. From penicillin 5,000,000 units per 10.0 cc., give penicillin 400,000 units.

5. How will you give 20 units of insulin from a vial labeled "Isophane Insulin Suspension U40"? You have a 2.0 cc. hypodermic syringe to use.

6. How many minims of regular insulin U100 will be needed to give 60 units?

7. Your patient has been on 40 units of regular insulin U40 and has several vials of this strength insulin. His order has been changed to 60 units of regular insulin. How will you measure this amount in a 2.0 cc. hypodermic syringe using the insulin he has on hand?

8. How much Lente insulin U80 will be needed to give 64 units?

**SEE OTHER SIDE
FOR ANSWERS**

ANSWERS TO PROBLEMS ON PAGE 60
DRUGS MEASURED IN UNITS

1. $\dfrac{DU}{HU} = \dfrac{5,000 \text{ units}}{20,000 \text{ units/ml.}} =$

   $\dfrac{5}{20/\text{ml.}} = $ 0.25 ml. of Heparin sodium solution containing 20,000 units per ml. will be needed to give 5,000 units of heparin sodium.

2. 10.0 ml. = 1,000,000 units
   1.0 ml. = 100,000 units

   $\dfrac{DU}{HU} = \dfrac{50,000 \text{ units}}{100,000 \text{ units/ml.}} =$

   $\dfrac{5}{10/\text{ml.}} = $ 0.5 ml. of penicillin G solution containing 1,000,000 units per 10.0 ml. will be needed to give 50,000 units of penicillin G.

3. 5.0 ml. = 3,000,000 units
   1.0 ml. = 600,000 units

   $\dfrac{DU}{HU} = \dfrac{600,000 \text{ units}}{600,000 \text{ units/ml.}} =$

   $\dfrac{6}{6/\text{ml.}} = $ 1.0 ml. of penicillin solution labeled 3,000,000 units per 5.0 ml. will be needed in order to give 600,000 units of penicillin.

4. 10.0 cc. = 5,000,000 units
   1.0 cc. = 500,000 units

   $\dfrac{DU}{HU} = \dfrac{400,000 \text{ units}}{500,000 \text{ units/cc.}} =$

   $\dfrac{4}{5.0/\text{cc.}} = $ 0.8 cc. penicillin solution containing 5,000,000 units in 10.0 cc. will be needed in order to give 400,000 units of penicillin.

5. $\dfrac{DU}{HU} = \dfrac{20 \text{ units}}{40 \text{ units/cc.}} = \dfrac{2}{4/cc.} =$

$\dfrac{1}{2/cc.} = \underline{0.5 \text{ cc. of Isophane Insulin Suspension will be needed to give 20 units.}}$

6. $\dfrac{DU}{HU} = \dfrac{60 \text{ units}}{100 \text{ units/cc.}} = \dfrac{6}{10/cc.} = 0.6/cc.$

To change cc. to minims, multiply the number of cc. by 15.

$0.6/cc. \times 15 = \underline{9 \text{ minims of regular insulin U100 will be needed to give 60 units.}}$

7. $\dfrac{DU}{HU} = \dfrac{60 \text{ units}}{40 \text{ units/cc.}} = \dfrac{6}{4/cc.} = \dfrac{3}{2/cc.} =$

$\underline{1.5 \text{ cc. of regular insulin U40 must be measured to give 60 units.}}$

8. $\dfrac{DU}{HU} = \dfrac{64 \text{ units}}{80 \text{ units/cc.}} = \dfrac{8}{10/cc.} =$

$\underline{0.8 \text{ cc. of Lente insulin U80 will be needed to give 64 units.}}$

9

Preparation of Drugs Packaged in Dry Form

Drugs that are unstable in solution may also be packaged in dry form in ampuls or vials. When you are ready to use the drug, you will dissolve the dry drug in the correct diluent. Information concerning the correct diluent will be packaged with the drug or may be obtained from the pharmacist or from pharmacology books.

The most common practice is to prepare the solution so that 1.0 cc. will contain the amount of the drug you wish to administer. When a multi-dose vial is used, the vial must be relabeled stating the amount of drug contained in each cubic centimeter of the fluid and the date the fluid was prepared.

The formula you will need to solve this type of problem is presented here. This formula will be used only when the amount of the drug does not increase the amount of the solution. When the drug increases the amount of the solution, specific directions as to the quantity of diluent will be packaged with the drug and must be followed explicitly.

	1. Certain drugs come from the pharmacy in dry powder form in a vial. The vial may contain the quantity of drug required for a single injection or may contain enough medication for several _____ .

1. doses (or injections)	2. In a single dose vial the amount of diluent used is usually 1.0 to 2.0 cc. However, the nurse should check the accompanying literature to determine the optimum _____ and kind of diluent for that particular preparation.
2. volume (or amount)	3. In the multiple-dose vial it is usually desirable to dissolve the drug in a volume of diluent necessary to make 1.0 cc. of the solution equivalent to the desired _____ .
3. dose	4. The proportion formula to determine the amount of diluent needed is: $$\frac{\text{Desired units}}{\text{Units on Hand}} = \frac{\text{Desired volume}}{x \text{ volume}}$$ According to frame #3, the Desired volume is usually _____ . x volume is the amount of diluent which will be added to the dry drug.
4. 1.0 cc.	5. Example: The label on a vial of powdered penicillin reads: "Penicillin. 1,000,000 U.S.P. Units." The physician has ordered penicillin 100,000 units Stat. and b.i.d. How many cubic centimers of diluent will be needed to produce a solution containing 100,000 units per cc.? Use formula from frame #4. $$\frac{DU}{HU} = \frac{V}{x}$$ Substitute values: $$\frac{100{,}000 \text{ units}}{1{,}000{,}000 \text{ units}} = \frac{}{x}$$

5. 1.0 cc.	6. $\dfrac{100{,}000 \text{ units}}{1{,}000{,}000 \text{ units}} = \dfrac{1.0 \text{ cc.}}{x}$ 100,000 : 1,000,000 : : 1.0 cc. : x 100,000 x = 1,000,000.0 cc. x = _____
6. <u>10.0 cc. of diluent will be needed to produce a penicillin solution of 100,000 units/cc.</u>	7. After the nurse has added the diluent to the vial she must always label the vials as to the number of units contained in each _____.
7. cc.	8. Another example: How much diluent will be needed to make a solution of 100,000 units per cc. if the vial contains 2,000,000 units of dry drug? $\dfrac{DU}{HU} = \dfrac{V}{x}$ $\dfrac{}{} = \dfrac{1.0 \text{ cc.}}{x}$
8. $\dfrac{100{,}000 \text{ units}}{2{,}000{,}000 \text{ units}}$	9. $\dfrac{100{,}000 \text{ units}}{2{,}000{,}000 \text{ units}} = \dfrac{1.0 \text{ cc.}}{x}$ 100,000 : 2,000,000 : : 1.0 cc. : x 100,000 x = 2,000,000.0 cc. x = _____
9. <u>20.0 cc. of diluent will be needed to make a solution of 100,000 units/cc.</u>	10. Some drugs may increase the volume of the solution. This formula can be used only when the volume of the dry drug does not increase the volume of the _____.
10. solution	11. When the dry drug increases the volume of the solution, specific instructions will be given by the manufacturer for the _____ of diluent to be used.

11. amount	12. Example: Streptomycin sulfate for injection. Given a vial containing 1.0 Gm. of the dry drug. Instructions: for 100.0 mg. per cc., add 9.2 cc. of diluent. The nurse will add 9.2 cc. of diluent to the dry drug, which will give a total of 10.0 cc. of solution where each cc. will contain _____ of the drug.
12. 100.0 mg.	13. How about some practice problems? We will use only problems in which the dry drug <u>does</u> <u>not</u> increase the volume of the solution.

PRACTICE PROBLEMS
DRUGS IN DRY FORM
(ANSWERS ON PAGE 68)

1. How much diluent will be required to prepare a solution of benzathine penicillin G of 500,000 units per cc. when the vial contains 1,000,000 units of the dry drug?

2. Given a vial containing 750 units of a drug in dry form, how will you prepare a solution containing 150 units per cc.?

3. How much diluent will be needed to give a solution of 25,000 units per cc. if the vial contains 200,000 units of dry drug?

4. A vial of potassium penicillin G contains 2,000,000 units of the dry drug. How much diluent will be needed to make a solution that contains 400,000 units per cc.?

ANSWERS TO PROBLEMS ON PAGE 67
DRUGS IN DRY FORM

1. $\dfrac{DU}{HU} = \dfrac{V}{x}$

   $\dfrac{500{,}000 \text{ units}}{1{,}000{,}000 \text{ units}} = \dfrac{1.0 \text{ cc.}}{x}$

   $500{,}000 : 1{,}000{,}000 :: 1.0 \text{ cc.} : x$

   $500{,}000\, x = 1{,}000{,}000.0 \text{ cc.}$

   $x = 2.0$ cc. diluent will be needed to prepare a solution of benzathine penicillin G 500,000 units per cc.

2. $\dfrac{DU}{HU} = \dfrac{V}{x}$

   $\dfrac{150 \text{ units}}{750 \text{ units}} = \dfrac{1.0 \text{ cc.}}{x}$

   $150 : 750 :: 1.0 \text{ cc.} : x$

   $150\, x = 750.0 \text{ cc.}$

   $x = 5.0$ cc. diluent will be needed to prepare a solution containing 150 units of drug per cc.

3. $\dfrac{DU}{HU} = \dfrac{V}{x}$

   $\dfrac{25{,}000 \text{ units}}{200{,}000 \text{ units}} = \dfrac{1.0 \text{ cc.}}{x}$

   $25{,}000 : 200{,}000 :: 1.0 \text{ cc.} : x$

   $25{,}000\, x = 200{,}000.0 \text{ cc.}$

   $x = 8.0$ cc. of diluent will be needed to prepare a solution containing 25,000 units of drug per cc.

4. $\dfrac{DU}{HU} = \dfrac{V}{x}$

   $\dfrac{400{,}000 \text{ units}}{2{,}000{,}000 \text{ units}} = \dfrac{1.0 \text{ cc.}}{x}$

   $400{,}000 : 2{,}000{,}000 :: 1.0 \text{ cc.} : x$

   $400{,}000\, x = 2{,}000{,}000.0 \text{ cc.}$

   $x = 5.0$ cc. diluent will be needed to prepare a solution containing 400,000 units of potassium penicillin G per cc.

10

Preparation of Solutions

In giving nursing care, you may need to prepare a solution or to teach someone else how to do it. Solutions are commonly used for such purposes as irrigations or soaks and, depending on the situation, may be sterile or unsterile. A solution is defined as a clear, homogeneous mixture which has no tendency to settle on standing. It is made by dissolving one or more substances in a liquid (the solvent). These substances (solutes) may be in the form of a gas, a liquid or a solid and may be the pure drug or the drug in a concentrated solution.

The strength of the solution is expressed in percentage or as a ratio. Percentage indicates the amount of the drug present in 100 parts of the solution. It is a fraction, the numerator of which is expressed, and the denominator understood to be 100; e.g., 25 per cent is 25/100. Ratio is another way of indicating the relationship between the amount of the drug and the amount of the solution; e.g., a 1:10 solution contains one part of the pure drug in ten parts of solution. Ratio and percentage really mean the same thing. For instance, at 25 per cent solution also can be expressed as a 1:4 solution. It is important to remember when working problems in percentage and ratio that all measurements be kept in the same system.

	1. When caring for her patients the nurse often will be called on to prepare a liquid mixture or solution for irrigations, soaks or other treatments. A liquid, homogeneous mixture consisting of two or more components is called a _____ .

69

1. solution	2. In most common solutions, one of the components is a liquid in which the other component is dissolved. This liquid portion is referred to as the solvent, and the component which is _____ in it is known as the solute. The solute may be either solid or liquid.
2. dissolved	3. The most commonly used solvent is water. In a sodium chloride solution, the solvent would be _____.
3. water	4. The solute in a sodium chloride solution would be _____.
4. sodium chloride	5. For a solution that need not be sterile (as a mouth wash), ordinary tap water is the _____ most frequently used.
5. solvent	6. To make a sterile solution (for use on a wound) the most common solvent would be _____ _____.
6. sterile water	7. Solutions are made from <u>pure drugs</u>, <u>tablets</u> or <u>stock solutions</u>. A pure drug is an unadulterated substance in solid or liquid form. Expressed in per cent, a pure drug is _____.
7. 100%	8. Tablets containing a known quantity of the pure drug may be used to make a solution. The _____ is essentially a preparation of the pure drug.
8. tablet	9. A stock solution is a relatively strong solution from which a weaker solution can be made. Stock solutions are usually _____ to make a weaker solution.

9. diluted	10. The strength of a solution may be expressed by <u>percentage</u> or <u>ratio</u>.
	Percentage indicates:
	  (a) the number of grains of the drug in 100 grains.
	  (b) the number of cc. of the drug in 100.0 cc. of solution.
	Thus: a 1% solution of cresol contains 1.0 cc. of cresol in _____ solution. (Cresol is a liquid.)

10. 100.0 cc.	11. In 200.0 cc. of a 1% solution of cresol, there are _____ of the pure drug.
11. 2.0 cc.	12. Ratio (when used with solutions) denotes the relative amounts of <u>solute</u> and <u>solvent</u>. Here, the metric system is almost invariably used. Thus: 1:1,000 indicates 1.0 Gm. or 1.0 cc. of pure drug in each 1,000.0 cc. of solution. 2:1,000 therefore indicates 2.0 Gm. (or 2.0 cc.) of _____ _____ in 1,000.0 cc. of solution.
12. pure drug	13. A solution labeled 1.0 ml. :1,000 ml. contains _____ solute in _____ solution.
13. 1.0 ml. 1,000.0 ml.	14. Now, let's work some problems together where the strength of the solution is expressed in percentage. The formula to be used is: $$\frac{\text{Desired \%}}{\text{On Hand \%}} = \frac{\text{quantity of solute (x)}}{\text{quantity of solution (V)}}$$ or $$\frac{D\%}{H\%} = \frac{x}{V}$$ This formula will be solved as an incomplete proportion. D% : H%: : _____ : _____

14. x V	15. Example: How many cc. of pure drug will be needed to prepare one liter of a 40% solution? How will you prepare the solution? $$\dfrac{D\%}{H\%} = \dfrac{x}{V}$$ Substitute known values: $$\dfrac{40\%}{\rule{1cm}{0.4pt}} = \dfrac{x}{1{,}000.0 \text{ cc. (1.0 liter)}}$$
15. 100%	16. $\dfrac{40\%}{100\%} = \dfrac{x}{1{,}000.0}$ cc. 40 : 100 : : _____
16. x : 1,000.0 cc.	17. 40 : 100 : : x : 1,000.0 cc. 100 x = 40,000.0 cc. x = _____
17. <u>400.0 cc. of pure drug will be needed.</u>	18. <u>To prepare the 40% solution of drug place the 400.0 cc. of pure drug, in a container and add water to make</u> _____ .
18. <u>1,000.0 cc.</u>	19. Example: Prepare 250.0 cc. of a 1% cresol solution. How much cresol will be needed? How will you prepare the solution? We will work together: $$\dfrac{D\%}{H\%} = \dfrac{x}{V}$$ $$\dfrac{1\%}{100\%} = \dfrac{\rule{1cm}{0.4pt}}{\rule{1cm}{0.4pt}}$$
19. $\dfrac{x}{250.0 \text{ cc.}}$	20. $\dfrac{1\%}{100\%} = \dfrac{x}{250.0 \text{ cc.}}$ 1 : 100 : : x : 250.0 cc. Finish calculations and label answer.

20. $100x = 250.0$ cc.

  $x = 2.5$ cc. of cresol will be needed. To this amount of drug add water to make 250.0 cc. of solution. This is a 1% cresol solution.

21. 5 : 100 :: 5.0 Gm. or cc. : x

  $5x = 500.0$ Gm. or cc.

  $x = 100.0$ cc.

  It is stated in the volume unit rather than solid unit. The 5.0 Gm. of neomycin sulfate is dissolved in 100.0 cc. of sterile water — 100.0 cc. of a 5% neomycin sulfate solution.

21. One more example:

  5.0 Gm. of neomycin sulfate for solution, sterile, is dispensed in a vial. How much 5% solution for wet dressings can be made from one vial?

  Note: In this problem, the amount of solute is known rather than the amount of solution to be made.

  The same basic formula is used:

  $$\frac{D\%}{H\%} = \frac{V}{x} \quad \text{(quantity of solute)} \atop \text{(quantity of solution)}$$

  $$\frac{5\%}{100\%} = \frac{5.0 \text{ Gm. or cc.}}{x}$$

  Finish calculations and label answer.

22. Are you ready for some practice problems? If so, go on and work the following. The answers will be found at the end of the chapter.

PRACTICE PROBLEMS
SOLUTIONS EXPRESSED IN PER CENT
(ANSWERS ON PAGES 78-79-80)

1. From a 3% hydrogen peroxide solution, how will you prepare one ounce of a 1% solution?

2. How will you make one quart of a 10% solution of Lysol?

3. How much chloramine-T (a liquid) will be needed to make two liters of a 2% solution?

4. How many cc. of 0.02% potassium permanganate solution can be made from 0.3 Gm. of potassium permanganate crystals?

5. How will you prepare one ounce of 5% argyrol for a bladder irrigation from a 20% solution?

6. How much 0.25% cresol solution can be made from 250.0 cc. of a 1% cresol solution?

7. How much 25% argyrol is needed to make eight ounces of 1:20 solution of argyrol?

8. How much 75% solution of alcohol will be required to make one pint of a 1:2 alcohol solution?

	23. When the strength of the solution is expressed in ratio, this formula will be used: $$\frac{\text{Desired Ratio}}{\text{On Hand Ratio}} = \frac{\text{quantity of solute}}{\text{quantity of solution}}$$ or $$\frac{DR}{HR} = \frac{\rule{1cm}{0.4pt}}{\rule{1cm}{0.4pt}}$$
23. $\frac{x}{V}$ Does this seem familiar?	24. Example: How much solute will be needed to make 2,000.0 ml. of a 1:5,000 bichloride of mercury solution from a 1:1,000 solution? Let's work together: $$\frac{DR}{HR} = \frac{x}{V}$$ $$\frac{1:5,000}{1:1,000} = \frac{\rule{1cm}{0.4pt}}{\rule{1cm}{0.4pt}}$$
24. $\frac{x}{2,000.0 \text{ ml.}}$	25. $\frac{1/5,000}{1/1,000} = \frac{x}{2,000.0 \text{ ml.}}$ $1/5,000 : 1/1,000 :: x : 2,000.0$ ml. $1/1,000\ x = 2,000.0$ ml. X $1/5,000$ $x = \rule{2cm}{0.4pt}$ Finish calculations and label answer.

25. $x = 2/5$ ml. $\div$ 1/1,000 $x = \underline{400.0 \text{ ml. of the}}$ <u>1/1,000 bichloride of mercury solution will be needed</u>. (Note: Here, the problem asks only how much drug will be needed.)	26. Example: How will you prepare one quart of 1:20 solution of boric acid from the crystals? $\dfrac{DR}{HR} = \dfrac{x}{V}$ $\dfrac{1/20}{1/1} = \dfrac{x}{1,000.0 \text{ cc.}}$ (This is the equivalent of 1 quart) $1/20 : 1/1 :: x : 1000.0$ cc. $1 x = 1,000.0$ cc. $\times$ 1/20 $x = \underline{\qquad}$ <u>of boric acid crystals will be needed. Add water to make</u> <u>solution. You now have one quart of 1:20 solution of boric acid.</u>
26. 50.0 Gms. 1,000.0 cc. (1 quart) Note: This problem asks how you will prepare the solution.)	27. Now, if you are ready, try the following practice problems. In solving any problems, always remember to <u>keep all measurements in the same system</u>.

PRACTICE PROBLEMS
SOLUTIONS EXPRESSED IN RATIO
(ANSWERS ON PAGES 81-82-83)

1. How will you make 200.0 ml. of 1:40 phenol solution from a 1:20 phenol solution?

2. Prepare 1,000.0 cc. of 1:5,000 solution of potassium permanganate from a 1:500 solution.

3. Make one gallon of 5% phenol solution from a 1:5 phenol solution.

4. Prepare 50.0 cc. of a 10% solution of magnesium sulfate from a 1:2 magnesium sulfate solution.

5. How much 1:2,000 solution can be made from two 7 1/2 grain bichloride of mercury tablets?

6. How much stock solution of benzalkonium chloride 1:1,000 will be needed to make one liter of 1:10,000 solution?

7. How many 5 grain tablets are needed to prepare two liters of 1:6,000 potassium permanganate solution?

8. How will you prepare 300.0 cc. of 1:20,000 solution from a silver nitrate solution 1:1,000?

**SEE OTHER SIDE
FOR ANSWERS**

ANSWERS TO PROBLEMS ON PAGES 73-74
SOLUTIONS EXPRESSED IN PER CENT

1. $\dfrac{D\%}{H\%} = \dfrac{x}{V}$

    $\dfrac{1\%}{3\%} = \dfrac{x}{30.0 \text{ cc.}}$ (equivalent of 1 fluid ounce)

    $1 : 3 :: x : 30.0$ cc.

    $3x = 30.0$ cc.

    x = <u>10.0 cc. of 3% hydrogen peroxide solution will be needed. Add water to make 30.0 cc. (1 fluid ounce.) You now have one ounce of 1% hydrogen peroxide solution.</u>

2. $\dfrac{D\%}{H\%} = \dfrac{x}{V}$

    $\dfrac{10\%}{100\%} = \dfrac{x}{1,000.0 \text{ cc.}}$ (equivalent of 1 quart)

    $10 : 100 :: x : 1,000.0$ cc.

    $100 x = 10,000.0$ cc.

    x = <u>100.0 cc. Lysol will be needed. Add water to make 1,000.0 cc. (1 quart.) You now have one quart of 10% Lysol solution.</u>

3. $\dfrac{D\%}{H\%} = \dfrac{x}{V}$

    $\dfrac{2\%}{100\%} = \dfrac{x}{2,000.0 \text{ cc.}}$

    $2 : 100 :: x : 2,000.0$ cc.

    $100 x = 4,000.0$ cc.

    x = <u>40.0 cc. of chloramine-T will be needed. Add water to make 2,000.0 cc. You now have 2 liters of 2% chloramine-T solution.</u>

4. 1.0 Gm. = 1.0 cc.   0.3 Gm. = 0.3 cc.

$$\frac{D\%}{H\%} = \frac{V}{x}$$

$$\frac{0.02\%}{100\%} = \frac{0.3 \text{ cc.}}{x}$$

0.02 : 100 : : 0.3 cc. : x

0.02 x = 30.0 cc.

x = 1,500.0 cc. of 0.02% potassium permangante solution can be made from 0.3 Gm. potassium permanganate.

5. $$\frac{D\%}{H\%} = \frac{x}{V}$$

$$\frac{5\%}{20\%} = \frac{x}{30.0 \text{ cc. (equivalent of 1 ounce)}}$$

5 : 20 : : x : 30.0 cc.

20 x = 150.0 cc.

x = 7.5 cc. of the 20% argyrol solution will be needed. Add water to make 30.0 cc. (1 ounce). You now have one ounce of 5% argyrol solution.

6. $$\frac{D\%}{H\%} = \frac{V}{x}$$

$$\frac{0.25\%}{1\%} = \frac{250.0 \text{ cc.}}{x}$$

0.25 : 1 : : 250.0 cc. : x

0.25 x = 250.0 cc.

x = 1,000.0 cc. of 0.25% cresol solution can be made from 250.0 cc. of 1% cresol solution.

7. Change 1:20 to its per cent equivalent--5%

(1:20 = 1/20   1/20 X 100 = 5%   Do you need to review this process?)

$$\frac{D\%}{H\%} = \frac{x}{V}$$

$$\frac{5\%}{25\%} = \frac{x}{240.0 \text{ cc. (equivalent of 8 ounces)}}$$

5 : 25 : : x : 240.0 cc.

25 x = 1,200.0 cc.

x = 48.0 cc. of 25% argyrol is needed. Add water to make 240.0 cc. You now have eight ounces of 1:20 argyrol solution.

8. Change 1:2 to the per cent equivalent –50%

(1:2 = 1/2   1/2 X 100 = 50%)

$$\frac{D\%}{H\%} = \frac{x}{V}$$

$$\frac{50\%}{75\%} = \frac{x}{500.0 \text{ cc. (equivalent of 1 pint)}}$$

50 : 75 : : x : 500.0 cc.

75 x = 25,000.0 cc.

x = 333.33 cc. of 75% alcohol will be needed. (Round off to 333.0 cc.). Add water to make 500.0 cc. You now have one pint of 1:2 alcohol solution.

ANSWERS TO PROBLEMS ON PAGES 75-76
SOLUTIONS EXPRESSED IN RATIO

1. $\dfrac{DR}{HR} = \dfrac{x}{V}$

   $\dfrac{1/40}{1/20} = \dfrac{x}{200.0 \text{ ml.}}$

   $1/40 : 1/20 :: x : 200.0 \text{ ml.}$

   $1/20 \, x = 200.0 \text{ ml.} \times 1/40$

   x = <u>100.0 ml. of 1:20 phenol solution needed. Add water to make 200.0 ml. You now have 200.0 ml. of 1:40 phenol solution.</u>

2. $\dfrac{DR}{HR} = \dfrac{x}{V}$

   $\dfrac{1/5,000}{1/500} = \dfrac{x}{1,000.0 \text{ cc.}}$

   $1/5,000 : 1/500 :: x : 1,000.0 \text{ cc.}$

   $1/500 \, x = 1,000.0 \text{ cc.} \times 1/5,000$

   x = <u>100.0 cc. of 1/500 potassium permanganate solution is needed. Add water to make 1,000.0 cc. You now have 1,000.0 cc. of 1:5,000 solution of potassium permanganate.</u>

3. 1 gallon = 4,000.0 cc.

   Change 5% to its ratio equivalent 1:20

   (5% = 5/100 = 1/20 = 1:20. Do you need to review this process?)

   $\dfrac{DR}{HR} = \dfrac{x}{V}$

   $\dfrac{1/20}{1/5} = \dfrac{x}{4,000.0 \text{ cc.}}$

   $1/20 : 1/5 :: x : 4,000.0 \text{ cc.}$

   $1/5 \, x = 4,000.0 \text{ cc.} \times 1/20$

   x = <u>1,000.0 cc. of 1:5 phenol solution is needed. Add water to make 4,000.0 cc. (1 gallon). You now have one gallon of 5% phenol solution.</u>

4. Change 10% to its ratio equivalent 1:10

   (10% = 10/100 = 1/10 = 1:10)

   $$\frac{DR}{HR} = \frac{x}{V}$$

   $$\frac{1/10}{1/2} = \frac{x}{50.0 \text{ cc}}$$

   1/10 : 1/2 : : x : 50.0 cc.

   1/2 x = 50.0 cc. X 1/10

   x = <u>10.0 cc. of 1:2 magnesium sulfate solution is needed. Add water to make 50.0 cc. You now have 50.0 cc. of a 10% magnesium sulfate solution.</u>

5. Ratio indicates metric system; therefore, change grains to grams.
   gr. 7 1/2 x 2 = gr. 15 = 1.0 Gm.

   $$\frac{DR}{HR} = \frac{x}{V}$$ Remember where V is desired, 1.0 Gm. = 1.0 cc.

   $$\frac{1/2,000}{1/1} = \frac{1.0 \text{ Gm.}}{x}$$

   1/2,000 : 1/1 : : 1.0 Gm. : x

   1/2,000 x = 1.0 Gm.

   x = <u>2,000.0 cc. of 1:2,000 bichloride of mercury solution can be made from two tablets bichloride of mercury each gr. 7 1/2.</u>

6. $$\frac{DR}{HR} = \frac{x}{V}$$

   $$\frac{1/10,000}{1/1,000} = \frac{x}{1,000.0 \text{ cc.}}$$

   1/10,000 : 1/1,000 : : x : 1,000.0 cc.

   1/1,000 x = 1,000.0 cc X 1/10,000

   x = <u>100.0 cc. of 1:1,000 benzalkonium chloride solution will be needed.</u>

7. 5 grains = 0.3 Grams

$$\frac{DR}{HR} = \frac{x}{V}$$

$$\frac{1/6,000}{1/1} = \frac{x}{2,000.0 \text{ cc. (2 liters)}}$$

1/6,000 : 1/1 : : x : 2,000.0 cc.

x = 2,000.0 cc X 1/6,000

x = <u>0.3 Gm. (Since weight unit is desired, pure drug will be needed.) Therefore:</u>

$$\frac{D}{H} = \frac{0.3 \text{ Gm.}}{0.3 \text{ Gm.}} =$$ <u>1 potassium permanganate tablet 0.3 Gm. or 1 potassium permanganate tablet grains 5 will be needed.</u>

8. $$\frac{DR}{HR} = \frac{x}{V}$$

$$\frac{1/20,000}{1/1,000} = \frac{x}{300.0 \text{ cc.}}$$

1/20,000 : 1/1,000 : : x : 300.0 cc.

1/1,000 x = 300.0 cc. X 1/20,000

x = <u>15.0 cc. of 1:1,000 silver nitrate solution will be needed. Add water to make 300.0 cc. You now have 300.0 cc. of 1:20,000 silver nitrate solution.</u>

11

Medications for Infants and Children

Medications may be administered to infants and children by any of the routes used for adults. When administering medications to infants and children, the nurse will note that the amount of the drug given is <u>always less</u> than the usual adult dose. The amount to be given is calculated as a fractional part of the adult dose based on weight, age or body surface area. While the physician will state the amount of the drug he wishes the patient to have, it is important that the nurse be able to recognize an overdose, and it is her responsibility to insure that an overdose <u>not</u> be given.

In this chapter you will learn how to use the three formulas most commonly used to estimate the amount of a drug to be given to an infant or child. You will need to remember that these are used as guides only, and that the physiologic and pathologic condition of the patient will also influence the amount of medication given. In the determination of drug dosage, an individual over 12 is considered an adult; an individual between 2 and 12 is considered a child; and from birth to 24 months, the individual is considered an infant. The formula based on weight may also be used to determine the amount of a drug to be given to a very small adult.

	1. Nurses who work with infants and children will observe that the amount of a drug ordered is less than the usual adult dose. You will always question an order for an infant or child which is the _____ as the usual adult dose.
1. same	2. While the dose of the drug for an infant or child will be ordered by the physician, it is important that the nurse be able to recognize whether this dose is within safe _____.
2. limits (or range)	3. Several rules are used in current practice as guides to estimate the dose of drugs for infants and children. No one rule is completely satisfactory; therefore, these rules should be used only as a _____.
3. guide	4. The most accurate way to estimate the dose for an infant or child is by the use of body surface area. The physician will probably use the _____ _____ _____ of the patient to determine the amount of the drug he wishes the patient to have.
4. body surface area	Note: Body surface area is determined by the use of a nomogram. This is a method infrequently used by the the nurse; therefore, we refer you to a standard pediatrics textbook for information on the nomogram itself, its use, and the formulas involved.

	5. Rules which the nurse may use as a guide to estimate the correct dose for an infant or child are those based on the age or weight of the patient. If the age of the patient is known, you may use a rule based on _____ to calculate the dose.
5. age	6. Young's Rule is based on the age of the child. To estimate the dose of a drug for a 7-year-old boy the nurse could use _____ _____.
6. Young's Rule	7. Young's Rule states: $$\text{child's dose} = \frac{\text{age (in years)}}{\text{age (in years)} + 12} \times \text{adult dose}$$ Substitute the age of the boy in frame 6: $$\text{child's dose} = \frac{\rule{1cm}{0.4pt}}{\rule{1cm}{0.4pt} + 12} \times \text{adult dose}$$
7. $\dfrac{7 \text{ years}}{7 \text{ years}}$	8. Now we will work some problems together using Young's Rule. Example: If an adult receives Demerol 50.0 mg., how much Demerol would a 3-year-old child receive? $$\text{child's dose} = \frac{\text{age (in years)}}{\text{age (in years)} + 12} \times \text{adult dose}$$ Substitute in Young's Rule: $$\text{child's dose} = \frac{\rule{1cm}{0.4pt}}{\rule{1cm}{0.4pt}} \times \text{adult dose}$$
8. $\dfrac{3 \text{ years}}{3 \text{ years} + 12}$	9. $\text{child's dose} = \dfrac{3 \text{ years}}{3 \text{ years} + 12} \times 50.0$ mg. $x = \dfrac{3}{15} \times 50.0$ mg. $x = \rule{2cm}{0.4pt}$ Finish calculations and label answer.

9. $x = \frac{1}{5} \times 50.0$ mg. $x = \underline{10.0}$ $\underline{mg.}$ of $\underline{Demerol}$ $\underline{is}$ $\underline{this}$ $\underline{child's}$ $\underline{dose.}$	10. Example: An adult is receiving 0.5 Gm. streptomycin. How much streptomycin would a child of 4 years receive? child's dose = $\frac{\text{age (in years)}}{\text{age (in years)} + 12} \times$ adult dose Substitute values and complete calculations. Be sure to label your answer.
10. $x = \frac{4 \text{ years}}{4 \text{ years} + 12} \times 0.5$ Gm. $x = \frac{4}{16} \times 0.5$ Gm. $x = \frac{1}{4} \times 0.5$ Gm. $x = \underline{0.125}$ $\underline{Gm.}$ $\underline{streptomycin}$ $\underline{is}$ $\underline{this}$ $\underline{child's}$ $\underline{dose.}$	11. Following are some practice problems in which you may use Young's Rule.

PRACTICE PROBLEMS
YOUNG'S RULE
(ANSWERS ON PAGE 92)

1. If an adult receives tetracycline 250.0 mg. every 6 hours, how much tetracycline would a child of 8 years receive every 6 hours?

2. An average adult dose of atropine sulfate is gr. 1/150. How much atropine sulfate would you give to a 6-year-old child?

3. What would be a reasonable dosage of penicillin for a 3-year-old child if an adult is receiving penicillin 300,000 units twice a day?

	12. Fried's Rule (based on age) is used to estimate the dose of drugs for an infant. When the age of the infant is known the nurse may use ____ ____.
12. Fried's Rule	13. Fried's Rule states: infant's dose = $\dfrac{\text{age in months}}{150 \text{ months}}$ X adult dose Note: 150 months here indicates 12½ years (adult age). Substitute in the formula for an infant of 15 months where the usual adult dose is gr. 1. infant's dose = $\dfrac{\text{age in months}}{150 \text{ months}}$ X adult dose infant's dose = $\dfrac{\rule{1cm}{0.15mm}}{150 \text{ months}}$ X $\rule{1cm}{0.15mm}$
13. 15 months gr. 1	14. Let's solve the following problem again working step by step. Example: Determine the dosage of Gantrisin for a 15-month-old infant. Consider the adult dose of Gantrisin to be 0.5 Gm. infant's dose = $\dfrac{\text{age in months}}{150 \text{ months}}$ X adult dose Substitute values in Fried's Rule: x = $\dfrac{\rule{1cm}{0.15mm}}{\rule{1cm}{0.15mm}}$ X adult dose (0.5 Gm.)
14. $\dfrac{15 \text{ months}}{150 \text{ months}}$	15. x = $\dfrac{15 \text{ months}}{150 \text{ months}}$ X 0.5 Gm. x = $\rule{2cm}{0.15mm}$ Complete calculations and be sure to label your answer.

15. $\dfrac{15 \text{ months}}{150 \text{ months}}$ X

    0.5 Gm.

    $x = \dfrac{1}{10}$ X 0.5 Gm.

    x = <u>0.05 Gm. of</u>
    <u>Gantrisin</u> is
    this <u>infant's</u>
    <u>dose.</u>

16. Let's try another problem:

    If an adult receives morphine sulfate gr. 1/6, how much morphine sulfate should a 6-month-old infant receive?

    infant's dose = $\dfrac{\text{age in months}}{150 \text{ months}}$ X adult dose

    x = _____

    Substitute values in Fried's Rule; complete calculations, and label your answer.

16. $x = \dfrac{6 \text{ months}}{150 \text{ months}}$ X

    gr. 1/6

    $x = \dfrac{1}{150}$ X gr. $\dfrac{1}{1}$

    x = gr. <u>1/150</u> is
    this <u>infant's</u>
    <u>dose</u> of <u>morphine</u>
    <u>sulfate.</u>

17. Are you ready for some practice problems using Fried's Rule? If so, try the following.

PRACTICE PROBLEMS
FRIED'S RULE
(ANSWERS ON PAGE 93)

1. What is the dosage of Nembutal for a 5-month-old infant if the adult dosage is 90.0 mg.?

2. An adult receives 300,000 units of penicillin twice a day. How much penicillin would be reasonable dosage for a 10-month-old infant to receive twice a day?

3. If an adult is receiving Gantrisin 0.5 Gm., how much Gantrisin would an infant of 6 months receive?

	18. Doses based on the age of the child have definite limitations when the weight of the child varies greatly from 'normal.' <u>Clark's</u> <u>Rule</u> utilizes the relationship between the weight of the child and the weight of the average adult in estimating the drug dose. On the basis of weight (in this case for a child who weighs 60 pounds) the nurse may use _____ _____ to estimate the dose for the child.
18. Clark's Rule	19. Clark's Rule states: child's dose = $\dfrac{\text{weight in pounds}}{150 \text{ pounds(avg. adult)}}$ X adult dose Substitute for the child in the preceding frame. child's dose = $\dfrac{\overline{}}{150 \text{ pounds}}$ X adult dose
19. 60 pounds	20. Working step by step together, let's try this problem. Example: An adult receives aspirin gr. x. How many grains of aspirin would you give to a child weighing 45 pounds? child's dose = $\dfrac{\text{weight in pounds}}{150 \text{ pounds}}$ X adult dose x = $\dfrac{\overline{}}{\overline{}}$ X gr. 10 (Substitute values)
20. $\dfrac{45 \text{ pounds}}{150 \text{ pounds}}$	21. x = $\dfrac{45 \text{ pounds}}{150 \text{ pounds}}$ X gr. 10 x = _____ Finish solving the problem.

21. $x = \dfrac{45 \text{ pounds}}{150 \text{ pounds}} \times$ gr. 10 $x = \dfrac{3}{10} \times$ gr. 10 $x = \underline{\text{gr. iii of aspirin}}$ $\underline{\text{would}}$ $\underline{\text{be}}$ $\underline{\text{given}}$ $\underline{\text{to this}}$ $\underline{\text{child.}}$	22. Another example: If an adult receives Benadryl 50.0 mg., how much Benadryl would a child weighing 27 pounds receive? child's dose = $\dfrac{\text{weight in pounds}}{150 \text{ pounds}} \times$ adult dose Substitute values in Clark's Rule and complete the problem. $x = \underline{\hspace{2cm}} \times \underline{\hspace{1cm}}$
22. $x = \dfrac{27 \text{ pounds}}{150 \text{ pounds}} \times$ 50.0 mg. $x = \dfrac{27}{3} \times 1.0$ mg. $x = \underline{9.0 \text{ mg. of}}$ $\underline{\text{Benadryl}}$ $\underline{\text{would}}$ $\underline{\text{be}}$ $\underline{\text{given}}$ $\underline{\text{to this}}$ $\underline{\text{child.}}$	23. Now try some practice problems using Clark's Rule.

PRACTICE PROBLEMS
CLARK'S RULE
(ANSWERS ON PAGE 94)

1. What is the dosage of Terramycin for a child weighing 30 pounds if an adult is receiving Terramycin 100.0 mg.?

2. An adult is receiving 300,000 units of penicillin twice a day. How much penicillin would a child weighing 75 pounds receive twice a day?

3. An adult receives atropine sulfate gr. 1/150. How much atropine sulfate would a child weighing 90 pounds receive?

ANSWERS TO PROBLEMS ON PAGE 87
YOUNG'S RULE

1. Child's dose = $\dfrac{\text{age (in years)}}{\text{age (in years)} + 12}$ X adult dose

   $x = \dfrac{8 \text{ years}}{8 \text{ years} + 12}$ X 250.0 mg.

   $x = \dfrac{8}{20}$ X 250.0 mg.

   $x = \dfrac{2}{5}$ X 250.0 mg.

   $x = \dfrac{2}{1}$ X 50.0 mg.

   x = <u>100.0 mg. of tetracycline is this child's dose.</u>

2. Child's dose = $\dfrac{\text{age (in years)}}{\text{age (in years)} + 12}$ X adult dose

   $x = \dfrac{6 \text{ years}}{6 \text{ years} + 12}$ X gr. 1/150

   $x = \dfrac{6}{18}$ X gr. 1/150

   $x = \dfrac{1}{3}$ X gr. 1/150

   x = <u>gr. 1/450 of atropine sulfate is this child's dose.</u>

3. Child's dose = $\dfrac{\text{age (in years)}}{\text{age (in years)} + 12}$ X adult dose

   $x = \dfrac{3 \text{ years}}{3 \text{ years} + 12}$ X 300,000 u.

   $x = \dfrac{3}{15}$ X 300,000 u.

   $x = \dfrac{1}{5}$ X 300,000 u.

   x = <u>60,000 u. of penicillin would be a reasonable child's dose.</u>

ANSWERS TO PROBLEMS ON PAGE 89
FRIED'S RULE

1. Infant's dose = $\dfrac{\text{age in months}}{150 \text{ months}}$ X adult dose

   $x = \dfrac{5 \text{ months}}{150 \text{ months}}$ X 90.0 mg.

   $x = \dfrac{1}{30}$ X 90.0 mg.

   x = <u>3.0 mg. of Nembutal is this infant's dose.</u>

2. Infant's dose = $\dfrac{\text{age in months}}{150 \text{ months}}$ X adult dose

   $x = \dfrac{10 \text{ months}}{150 \text{ months}}$ X 300,000 u.

   $x = \dfrac{1}{15}$ X 300,000 u.

   x = <u>20,000 units of penicillin would be this infant's dose.</u>

3. Infant's dose = $\dfrac{\text{age in months}}{150 \text{ months}}$ X adult dose

   $x = \dfrac{6 \text{ months}}{150 \text{ months}}$ X 0.5 Gm.

   $x = \dfrac{1}{25}$ X 0.5 Gm.

   x = <u>0.02 Gm. or 20.0 mg. of Gantrisin would be the infant dose.</u>

ANSWERS TO PROBLEMS ON PAGE 91
CLARK'S RULE

1. Child's dose = $\dfrac{\text{weight in pounds}}{150 \text{ pounds}}$ X adult dose

   $x = \dfrac{30 \text{ pounds}}{150 \text{ pounds}}$ X 100.0 mg.

   $x = \dfrac{1}{5}$ X 100.0 mg.

   $x =$ 20.0 mg. Terramycin would be this child's dose.

2. Child's dose = $\dfrac{\text{weight in pounds}}{150 \text{ pounds}}$ X adult dose

   $x = \dfrac{75 \text{ pounds}}{150 \text{ pounds}}$ X 300,000 u.

   $x = \dfrac{1}{2}$ X 300,000 u.

   $x =$ 150,000 units of penicillin would be given to this child twice a day.

3. Child's dose = $\dfrac{\text{weight in pounds}}{150 \text{ pounds}}$ X adult dose

   $x = \dfrac{90 \text{ pounds}}{150 \text{ pounds}}$ X gr. 1/150

   $x = \dfrac{3}{5}$ X gr. 1/150

   $x = \dfrac{1}{5}$ X gr. 1/50

   $x =$ gr. 1/250 of atropine sulfate would be this child's dose.

Comprehensive Examination
(ANSWERS ON PAGE 109)

Directions: Determine the correct answer and place the letter of your answer in the space provided.

1. 60.0 Kg. = ___?___ Gm.

    a. 0.006 Gm.
    b. 0.06 Gm.
    c. 600.0 Gm.
    d. 6,000.0 Gm.
    (e.) 60,000.0 Gm.

2. 75.0 mg. = ___?___ Gm.

    a. 7,500.0 Gm.
    b. 750.0 Gm.
    c. 0.75 Gm.
    (d.) 0.075 Gm.
    e. 0.0075 Gm.

3. 25.0 ml. = ___?___ cc.

    a. 2.5 cc.
    (b.) 25.0 cc.
    c. 250.0 cc.
    d. 500.0 cc.
    e. 2,500.0 cc.

4. 55.0 L. = ___?___ ml.

    a. 0.055 ml.
    b. 0.05 ml.
    c. 0.5 ml.
    d. 5,500.0 ml.
    (e.) 55,000.0 ml.

5. In the apothecaries' system, fifteen and one-half grains is written as

    a. 15 1/2 grains
    b. grains 15 1/2
    c. xv 1/2 grains
    (d.) grains xv$\overline{ss}$
    e. none of the above

96

6. drams (℥) vi = minims (m) __?__ .

    a. 40 m.
    b. 120 m.
    c. 230 m.
    d. 360 m.
    e. 400 m.

7. ounces (℥) 8 = drams __?__ .

    a. 24 drams
    b. 36 drams
    c. 48 drams
    d. 52 drams
    e. 64 drams

8. ounces 48 = pints __?__ .

    a. 2 pints
    b. 3 pints
    c. 4 pints
    d. 6 pints
    e. 7 pints

9. quarts 10 = pints __?__ .

    a. 5 pints
    b. 15 pints
    c. 20 pints
    d. 25 pints
    e. 30 pints

10. 240 drops = __?__ teaspoonful(s).

    a. 1 teaspoonful
    b. 2 teaspoonfuls
    c. 3 teaspoonfuls
    d. 4 teaspoonfuls
    e. 5 teaspoonfuls

11. 5 tablespoonfuls = __?__ teaspoonfuls.

    a. 10 teaspoonfuls
    b. 15 teaspoonfuls
    c. 20 teaspoonfuls
    d. 25 teaspoonfuls
    e. 30 teaspoonfuls

12. 3 ounces = ___?___ tablespoonfuls.

    a. 2 tablespoonfuls
    b. 4 tablespoonfuls
    c. 6 tablespoonfuls ⓒ
    d. 8 tablespoonfuls
    e. 10 tablespoonfuls

13. 5.0 Gm. = gr. ___?___.

    a. gr. 15
    b. gr. 30
    c. gr. 45
    d. gr. 60
    e. gr. 75 ⓔ

14. gr. viiss ___?___ Gm.

    a. 0.025 Gm.
    b. 0.5 Gm. ⓑ
    c. 0.75 Gm.
    d. 1.0 Gm.
    e. 2.5 Gm.

15. 180.0 Gm. = ounces (oz.) ___?___.

    a. 6 oz. ⓐ
    b. 10 oz.
    c. 250 oz.
    d. 540 oz.
    e. 5,400 oz.

16. ℥ xxx = ___?___ cc.

    a. 90 cc.
    b. 260 cc.
    c. 500 cc.
    d. 750 cc.
    e. 900 cc. ⓔ

17. 4.2 cc. = m. ___?___.

    a. 23 m.
    b. 40 m.
    c. 48 m.
    d. 60 m
    e. 63 m. ⓔ

18. You are to administer codeine sulfate gr. $\overline{ss}$. The tablets you have are labeled codeine sulfate 30.0 mg. How many tablet(s) will you administer?

   a. 1/2 tablet
   b. 1 tablet
   c. 1 1/2 tablets
   d. 2 tablets
   e. 2 1/2 tablets _____

19. You are to administer gantrisin 1.0 Gm. The tablets you have are labeled gantrisin 0.5 Gm. How many tablet(s) will you administer?

   a. 1/2 tablet
   b. 1 tablet
   c. 1 1/2 tablet
   d. 2 tablets
   e. 2 1/2 tablets _____

20. You are to administer phenobarbital 90.0 mg. The tablets you have are labeled phenobarbital gr. $\overline{ss}$. How many tablet(s) will you administer?

   a. 1 tablet
   b. 2 tablets
   c. 3 tablets
   d. 4 tablets
   e. 5 tablets _____

21. You are at home with an oral medication bottle labeled "Elixir of Donnatol ℥ i = gr. xv." Your doctor ordered you to take gr. xxx. How many teaspoonful(s) will you take?

   a. 1/2 teaspoonful
   b. 1 teaspoonful
   c. 2 teaspoonfuls
   d. 3 teaspoonfuls
   e. 3 1/2 teaspoonfuls _____

22. You have a bottle labeled "Elixir of Phenobarbital gr. xv/cc." You are to administer 0.5 Gm. orally. How many cc. do you prepare?

   a. 0.5 cc.
   b. 1 cc.
   c. 2 cc.
   d. 3 cc.
   e. 3.5 cc. _____

23. You are to give acetysalicylic acid gr. x. You have acetysalicylic acid tablets gr. iiss. How many tablet(s) do you need?

   a. 0.25 tablet
   b. 1.5 tablets
   c. 2.25 tablets
   d. 3.5 tablets
   (e.) 4.0 tablets _____

24. You are to give sulfasuxidine 2.0 Gm. The tablets you have are labeled sulfasuxidine gr. viiss. How many tablet(s) will you give?

   a. 0.25 tablet
   b. 1.0 tablet
   c. 2.25 tablets
   d. 3.0 tablets
   (e.) 4.0 tablets _____

25. You are to give aspirin gr. v. The tablets you have are labeled aspirin 0.3 Gm. How many tablet(s) will you give?

   a. 1/2 tablet
   (b.) 1 tablet
   c. 1 1/2 tablets
   d. 2 tablets
   e. 5 tablets _____

26. You are to give Milk of Magnesia ℥ i. How many cc's is this?

   a. 10 cc.
   b. 15 cc.
   c. 20 cc.
   d. 25 cc.
   (e.) 30 cc. _____

27. You are to drink 1,000 cc. of water in 8 hours. How many quart(s) (qt.) would this be?

   a. 1/2 qt.
   (b.) 1 qt.
   c. 1 1/2 qt.
   d. 2 qt.
   e. 2 1/2 qt. _____

28. You are to administer cascara ℥ i. How many teaspoonful(s) would this be?

    a. 1/2 teaspoonful
    (b.) 1 teaspoonful
    c. 1 1/2 teaspoonfuls
    d. 2 teaspoonfuls
    e. 2 1/2 teaspoonfuls   _____

29. You are to give digitalis leaf gr. $\overline{iss}$. The tablets you have are labeled 60 mg. How many tablet(s) will you give?

    a. 1/2 tablet
    b. 1 tablet
    (c.) 1 1/2 tablets
    d. 2 tablets
    e. 2 1/2 tablets   _____

30. You are to administer penicillin 750,000 units intramuscularly. The bottle of penicillin is labeled 300,000 units/cc. How many cc. will you administer?

    a. 0.4 cc.
    b. 0.8 cc.
    c. 1.5 cc.
    (d.) 2.5 cc.
    e. 3.5 cc.   _____

31. You are to administer morphine sulfate gr. 1/6 by injection. The supply of morphine sulfate tablets is labeled gr. 1/4. How many tablet(s) will you use?

    a. 1/3 tablet
    (b.) 2/3 tablet
    c. 1 tablet
    d. 1 1/3 tablets
    e. 1 1/2 tablets   _____

32. You are to give codeine phosphate gr. 1/3 by injection. You have a bottle of hypodermic tablets labeled codeine phosphate gr. 1/6. How many tablet(s) will you need to use?

    a. 1/2 tablet
    b. 1 1/2 tablets
    (c.) 2 tablets
    d. 2 1/2 tablets
    e. 4 tablets   _____

33. What quantity of diluent should be used to dissolve the tablets of codeine phosphate you need in problem 32?

   a. 5 minims
   b. 15 minims
   c. 5.0 cc.
   d. 15.0 ml.
   e. ℨ xx   _____

34. You have on hand hypodermic tablets labeled morphine sulfate 10.0 mg. You are to administer morphine sulfate 5.0 mg. How many tablet(s) will you need to use?

   a. 1/3 tablet
   b. 1/2 tablet
   c. 1 1/4 tablets
   d. 1 1/2 tablets
   e. 1 3/4 tablets   _____

35. If you dissolve the number of whole tablet(s) needed in problem 34 in 20 minims of sterile water, how many minims of this solution is equivalent to 5.0 mg. of morphine sulfate?

   a. 5 minims
   b. 8 minims
   c. 10 minims
   d. 15 minims
   e. 20 minims   _____

36. You have a terramycin solution containing 500.0 mg. in 1.0 cc. You are to give 400.0 mg. How much solution will you give?

   a. 0.2 cc.
   b. 0.5 cc.
   c. 0.8 cc.
   d. 1.25 cc.
   e. 1.55 cc   _____

37. You have a solution of cortisone acetate containing 25.0 mg. in 1.0 cc. You are to give 60.0 mg. How much solution will you give?

   a. 0.4 cc.
   b. 0.8 cc.
   c. 1.8 cc.
   d. 2.4 cc.
   e. 3.2 cc.   _____

38. You are to give 20 units of regular insulin. You have on hand a bottle labeled regular insulin U40 and a 2.0 cc. hypodermic syringe. How much solution will you give?

   a. 0.2 cc.
   (b.) 0.5 cc.
   c. 1.2 cc.
   d. 1.5 cc.
   e. 2.0 cc. _____

39. You are to give caffeine sodium benzoate gr. viiss. You have an ampul labeled "Caffeine Sodium Benzoate 0.5 Gm. in 2.0 cc." How much of this solution will you use?

   a. 0.2 cc.
   b. 0.5 cc.
   c. 1.2 cc.
   d. 1.5 cc.
   (e.) 2.0 cc. _____

40. You are to give 100,000 units of sodium penicillin G from a multiple-dose vial labeled "Sodium Penicillin G, 1,000,000 units per 10.0 cc." How many cc. will you need to use?

   (a.) 1.0 cc.
   b. 2.0 cc.
   c. 5.0 cc.
   d. 7.0 cc.
   e. 10.0 cc. _____

41. You are to give atropine sulfate 0.3 mg. You have a bottle labeled "Atropine Sulfate gr. 1/150 per cc." How much solution do you need to use?

   a. 0.5 cc.
   (b.) 0.75 cc.
   c. 1.0 cc.
   d. 1.5 cc.
   e. 1.75 cc. _____

42. You are to give chlorpromazine 0.075 Gm. from a bottle labeled chlorpromazine 25.0 mg. per ml. How much solution will you use?

   a. 1.5 ml.
   b. 2.0 ml.
   (c.) 3.0 ml.
   d. 3.5 ml.
   e. 4.0 ml. _____

43. You are to give atropine sulfate gr. 1/300. You have a bottle of solution labeled "Atropine Sulfate 0.4 mg. per cc." How much solution will you use?

   a. 0.5 cc.
   b. 1.0 cc.
   c. 1.5 cc.
   d. 2.0 cc.
   e. 2.5 cc.

44. You are to give 600,000 units of penicillin. You have a bottle labeled "Penicillin 3,000,000 units per 10.0 cc." How much solution will you use?

   a. 0.5 cc.
   b. 1.2 cc.
   c. 1.5 cc.
   d. 2.0 cc.
   e. 2.5 cc.

45. You have a vial containing 500 units of a drug in dry form. How much diluent will you use to prepare a solution containing 125 units of drug per cc.?

   a. 0.25 cc.
   b. 1.0 cc.
   c. 2.5 cc.
   d. 4.0 cc.
   e. 10.0 cc.

46. A vial of potassium penicillin G contains 3,000,000 units of the dry drug. How much diluent will be needed to make a solution that contains 400,000 units of this drug per cc.?

   a. 0.25 cc.
   b. 2.5 cc.
   c. 5.0 cc.
   d. 6.5 cc.
   e. 7.5 cc.

47. You have a vial containing 25.0 mg. of a drug in dry form. How much diluent will you use to prepare a solution containing 2.0 mg. of drug per cc.?

   a. 5.0 cc.
   b. 7.5 cc.
   c. 10.0 cc.
   d. 12.5 cc.
   e. 15.0 cc.

48. You are at home and need to prepare 8 oz. of a normal saline solution. (0.9% strength). How many teaspoonful(s) of table salt will you add to 8 oz. of hot water?

   a. 1/2 teaspoonful
   b. 1 teaspoonful
   c. 2 teaspoonfuls
   d. 2 1/2 teaspoonfuls
   e. 3 teaspoonfuls

49. You are to prepare 1,000.0 cc. of 1:5,000 solution of potassium permanganate. You have a stock solution labeled potassium permanganate 1:1,000. How many cc. of this stock solution do you need?

   a. 100.0 cc.
   b. 200.0 cc.
   c. 300.0 cc.
   d. 400.0 cc.
   e. 500.0 cc.

50. How many cc. of diluent do you need to add to the stock solution in problem 49 in order to prepare the 1,000.0 cc. of 1:5,000 potassium permanganate solution?

   a. 900.0 cc.
   b. 800.0 cc.
   c. 700.0 cc.
   d. 600.0 cc.
   e. 500.0 cc.

51. If an adult received Demerol 75.0 mg., what would you consider an appropriate dose of Demerol for an infant 10 months old?

   a. 3.5 mg.
   b. 5.0 mg.
   c. 7.5 mg.
   d. 25.0 mg.
   e. 34.0 mg.

52. An adult is receiving tetracyline 250.0 mg., 4 times a day. Which of the following dosages would be considered a safe single dosage for a child weighing 30 pounds?

   a. 5.0 mg.
   b. 8.0 mg.
   c. 30.0 mg.
   d. 50.0 mg.
   e. 80.0 mg.

53. How much aspirin would you consider a safe dosage for a child of 4 years if an adult received aspirin gr. x?

   a. gr. iiss
   b. gr. iii
   c. gr. v
   d. gr. viii
   e. gr. x

ANSWERS TO THE COMPREHENSIVE EXAMINATION

1. e	19. d	37. d
2. d	20. c	38. b
3. b	21. c	39. e
4. e	22. a	40. a
5. d	23. e	41. b
6. d	24. e	42. c
7. e	25. b	43. a
8. b	26. e	44. d
9. c	27. b	45. d
10. d	28. b	46. e
11. c	29. c	47. d
12. c	30. d	48. a
13. e	31. b	49. b
14. b	32. c	50. b
15. a	33. b	51. b
16. e	34. b	52. d
17. e	35. c	53. a
18. b	36. c	

Parson Library
N. I. U.
De Kalb, Illinois